Pilates *for* Wimps

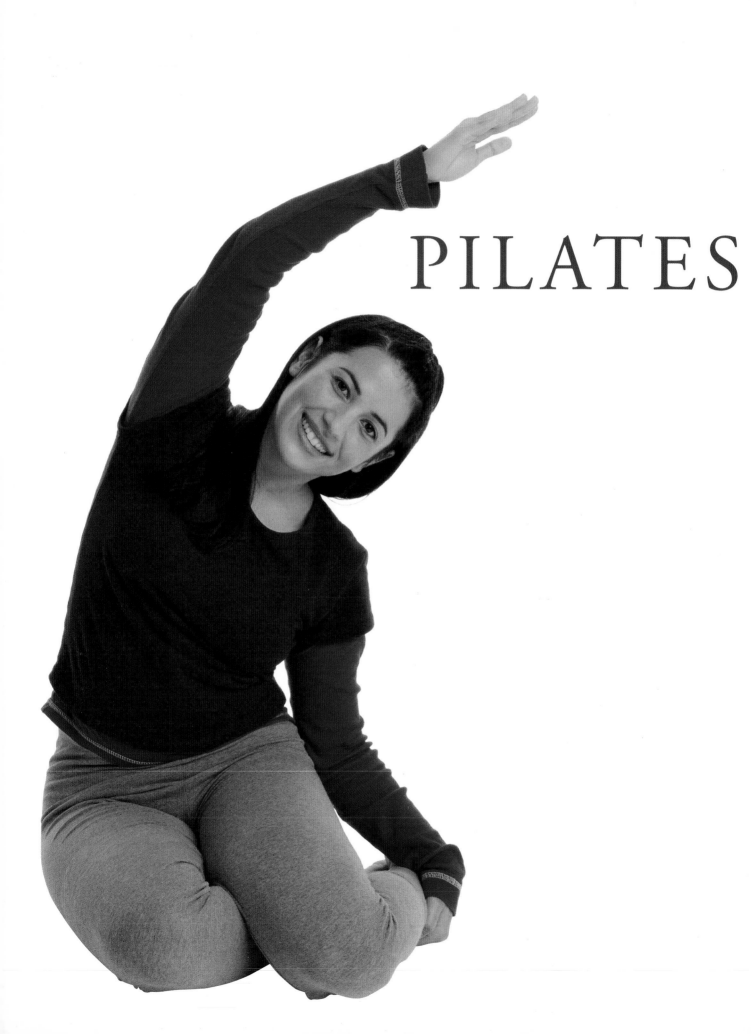

PILATES

for WIMPS

TOTAL FITNESS

FOR THE PARTIALLY

MOTIVATED

Jennifer DeLuca

Photography by Peter Murdoch

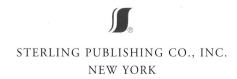

STERLING PUBLISHING CO., INC.
NEW YORK

For the teachers and students at BodyTonic

Design by Lubosh Cech *okodesignstudio.com*
Photography by Peter Murdoch
Illustration by Mona Mark
Models: Dayna Bealy; Fern Berenberg; Karen Brothers;
Bianca Craig; Jennifer De Luca; Dan Dome;
Marla Kochman; Gabrielle Nakash; Donald Porter;
Randy St. Louis

Library of Congress Cataloging-in-Publication Data Available

10 9 8 7 6 5 4 3 2 1
DeLuca, Jennifer
    Pilates for wimps : total fitness for the partially motivated / by
Jennifer DeLuca.
        p. cm.
    Includes index.
    ISBN 0-8069-9260-3
    1. Pilates method. 2. Physical fitness. 3. Exercise. I. Title.
RA781 .D413 2003
613. 7'1--dc22
                                2003014882
Published by Sterling Publishing Co., Inc.
387 Park Avenue South, New York, NY 10016
©2003 by Jennifer DeLuca
Distributed in Canada by Sterling Publishing
c/o Canadian Manda Group, One Atlantic Avenue, Suite 105
Toronto, Ontario, Canada M6K 3E7
Distributed in Great Britain by Chrysalis Books
64 Brewery Road, London N7 9 NT, England
Distributed in Australia by Capricorn Link (Australia) Pty. Ltd.
PO Box 704, Windsor, NSW 2756, Australia

Printed in China

Sterling ISBN 0-8069-9260-3

Acknowledgments

I would like to thank my inspirations, past, present, and future. I am forever grateful to have been in the classrooms of the great teachers in my life, Romana Kryzanowska Robert Mann, Bob Heath, Irene Dowd, Jackie Villamil. They are (or were) so obviously connected to the divine in their work. Witnessing them in their glow and experiencing their contagious enthusiasm for their crafts unearthed the joy of teaching within me. I owe the course of my life to them.

I have been filled with wonder and awe by the earliest devotees of the Pilates technique, many of whom I watched during my training at Drago's Gym. Seeing their bodies in action at 50-plus years young opened my eyes to the athleticism possible at any age. Romana, in the prime of her 70s, made a habit of hanging upside down in a split from the metal bars of the Cadillac. I have now made a promise to myself to perform a back walkover every year on my birthday. In my 80s, I hope I'll be looking at all of you upside down.

To my editor, Danielle Truscott, for the opportunity to put my knowledge to paper, and for busting out her cape in moments of chaos—"Thanks, Supergirl!"

Adam Rhynard and Michelle Ajami were kind enough to read this manuscript in the midst of its development. Their acute minds, unbounded curiosity, and constructive feedback contributed greatly to this project at a time when I needed it most. It is a beautiful thing to have people you trust and admire in your life.

My mom spotted me the cash for my first pieces of Pilates equipment. Big thanks go to her for that, in addition to raising me well with my dad. My parents imparted the values of compassion toward others, integrity in my work, and following my heart in all matters. I love wearing sweats to work every day.

In my present and my future, I owe my smiles and comfort to my husband, Tarik. Throughout the creation of this book and every moment in his presence, I have received great support and encouragement—this, along with his astounding sense of humor and staggering good looks, make me wonder if the joy in my life has any limits.

Special thanks, of course, go to the models in this book. I am honored and feel truly blessed to be associated with such a positive, adept, and sublimely pleasant group. It's a rarity to have a perfect ensemble for a project. You are all responsible for bringing this book to life, physically and spiritually. It could never have happened (and so smoothly, I might add!) without all of you.

Contents

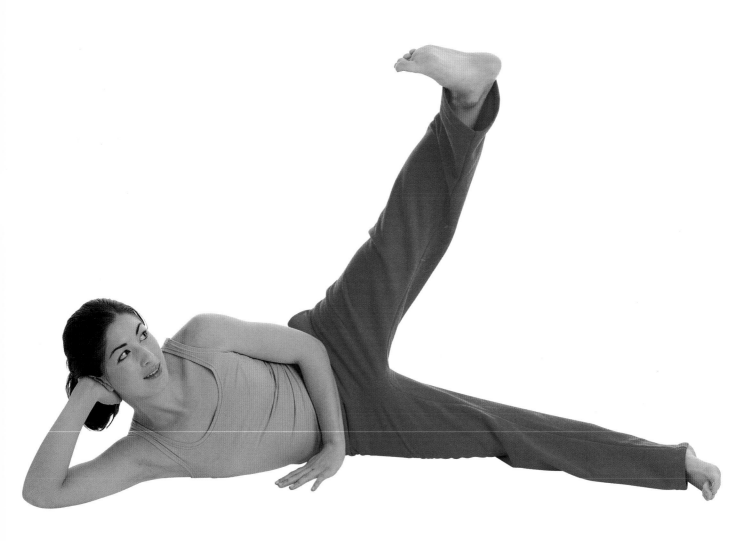

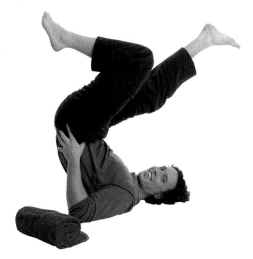

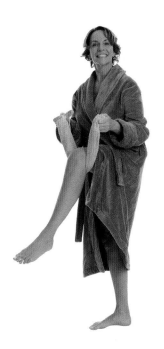

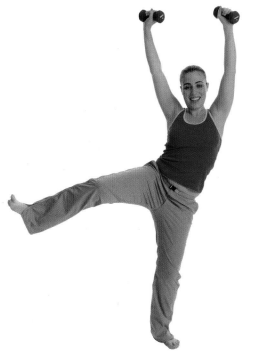

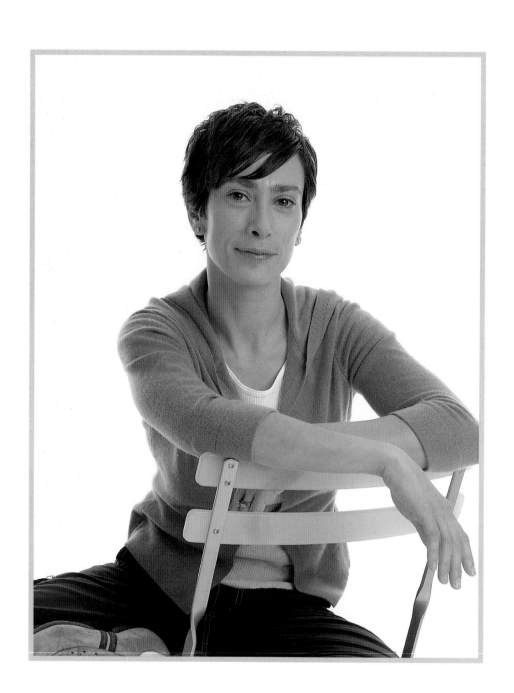

Author's Preface

Years ago, when I told people what I did for a living, they would say, "Pahlahteez? What's that? How do you spell it?" But not anymore. Pilates has grown in popularity at a rapid pace—and I'm not surprised. Oddly enough, the more out of shape you are, the more quickly you feel and see the benefits. It just takes one class. Throw the quintessential couch potato into a couple of classes, and that Pilates neophyte quickly becomes a fierce advocate for one of the most intelligent, engaging, efficient, and fun ways to exercise. The body changes quickly in posture, coordination, and muscle tone, creating an all-around healthier, happier, more agile person. So nowadays I hear a lot of "My sister does Pilates and swears by it!" or "Really? Wow. I've seen it at my gym and always wanted to try it out." And more and more I run into people who say, "Pilates! Where's your studio? I love Pilates! I'm an addict!"

Pilates first entered my life in 1985, when I had a semester of it as a student at the High School of Performing Arts in New York City. Our intense dance curriculum consisted of two hard-core dance classes a day, every day, for four years. Occasionally we had something like acting or stage makeup on the schedule . . . which meant 55 minutes of goofing off. But then they tossed in this *Pilates* class. To our dismay, this was not 55 minutes of pretending we were our favorite stuffed animal or playing with various shades of lip color. It was work. Luckily, it was just weird enough to keep us all engaged. The classical dance we studied strengthened our coordination and our limbs, but it didn't isolate postural problems, strengthen our abdominals, or eliminate "cheating." This is why the program directors chose Pilates. The simplicity of the technique freed us to focus on details of proper alignment that got lost in quick, complicated movements. We were able to learn more about our bodies, gain greater efficiency, and equalize our strength and flexibility. Plus, it was fun and felt good. The impression lasted, and years later Pilates became my saving grace.

Dance remained an integral part of my life throughout college and afterward as I danced for professional companies in New York City. When the financial struggle became too much to bear, I took a desk job. No more dancing. My physical world went from working barefoot and using muscle all day to wearing shoes and sitting at a computer. I just didn't feel like *me* anymore. My energy was miserably low, my neck was in knots, my lower back was weak, and I was irritable. The urge to fit something into my lunch hour that would make me feel stretched, strong, and energized—not compressed, exhausted and bored (which is what most commercial gyms had to offer)—became too great to ignore. As fate would have it, Drago's Gym, a Pilates studio that was home to Romana Kryzanowska, a direct descendant of Joseph Pilates, was just a few blocks away.

My new life was set in motion. Lunchtime workouts just twice a week transformed my body and revitalized my spirit. I felt long, powerful, and limber after every workout. People noticed that I had the "Pilates glow." I became an admitted addict of the technique, religiously taking two private sessions per week and practicing my Mat routine at home. My regular instructor at the time, Roxanne Murata, one of Romana's top protégés, was completely supportive when I told her I was considering the certification program: "You should definitely do it. It would be like a fish in water." I thank her today for that encouragement. In 1997 I completed my Pilates certification, and ever since then I've been confident that I do exactly what I am meant to do for a living.

The Pilates instructor's certificate went up on my wall, and my apartment was transformed into what looked like a jungle gym as I immediately began taking clients at my home in Park Slope, Brooklyn. My first private client was 50 years old and had extreme curvature in her lower back and hunched shoulders. After one month of Pilates, she eliminated the chiropractor from her list of weekly bills, and after a year, she had actually grown an inch and a quarter.

By then, along with my home clientele, I was teaching Pilates in Manhattan at JRW Physical Therapy, rehabilitating injuries along with the physical therapists, and leading lunchtime Pilates Mat classes at the offices of *People* magazine. The demand at my home studio had grown, too. Once-a-week clients were looking great, feeling more relaxed—they wanted to come twice a week. Their friends took notice and called for their own appointments. Their spouses were thrilled. For example, Marla's husband calls me Jennifer Pilates and has thanked me on many occasions for keeping his wife happy and fit. Paula started coming twice a week after her husband remarked, "Honey, you seem stressed today. When's your next Pilates session?" Perhaps the best thing my clients told me was "This

is the first form of exercise I've stuck with in my life!" (I still hear it all the time—and this is after four years and still going strong.) As much as I loved working at JRW and *People*, I decided to work with the people in my immediate community.

Today there's BodyTonic, Brooklyn's first full-service Pilates studio. It was very exciting when I opened in 1999, welcoming all those newcomers with fresh new bodies to work with. Some of them hadn't exercised in years. Some had gym memberships going to waste. Some came on the recommendation of a doctor or chiropractor. And some were avid athletes—runners, bladers, bikers, tennis players—seeking something different. Very few of them had actually studied Pilates, so I guess you could say 99 percent of the clientele that year were Pilates wimps.

There were a lot of basic level classes on the schedule at first, but the need for intermediate classes quickly appeared. So many people were coming regularly and improving! It was so moving to see the fruits of Joe's genius shining in the students' bodies. Debra, Susan, SJ, Lane, Dana, and countless others were kicking off their shoes and stretching long on their mats. And the changes they had made, not only in their muscle tone but also in the strength, grace, and freedom of their movements, the looks in their eyes, even in the ways they related to each other—it gave me goose bumps!

When I was approached to do this book, I was thrilled. This experience of working through the beginning with newcomers is fun. It's especially inspiring to work with people who have always *hated* exercise. I believe that human beings like to be physical. What leads a former slouch to a Pilates addiction? It feels good—it's interesting, progressive, diverse, and concise. It engages the mind, and the results are felt and seen immediately. To experience the body and mind working together and making progress is empowering. It's been a pleasure to see Pilates move previously unathletic people to take on new forms of fitness, such as skiing, tennis, or ballroom dancing, because they no longer feel klutzy and awkward. And I've seen that this transcends different personalities, limitations, interests, and ages. Even the models in this book are in different phases of their training. From novice to pro, and all with different bodies, lifestyles, and goals, Pilates has made their bodies, and their lives, better.

I love hearing people say "I can't believe I just did that!" And I'm incredibly excited to bring Pilates to anyone who might be starting out as a Pilates wimp.

What Is a Pilates Wimp?

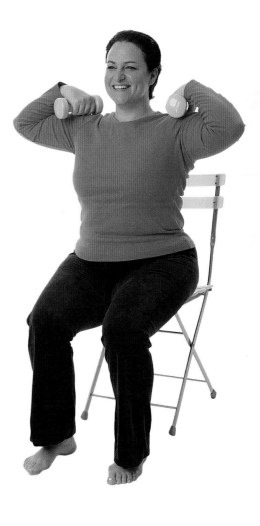

You could be a Pilates wimp if:

- You think of lab rats every time you see a room full of people on treadmills.

- You're sure that nothing (nothing!) could be more boring than running in place indoors.

- In a previous step aerobics class you crashed into your neighbor and were gently encouraged to take up swimming.

- You dislike, perhaps detest and aggressively avoid, "ab exercises."

- You're curious about Pilates because you've heard it's done lying down.

- You don't want to admit you're curious about Pilates, because your mom does it.

- You don't want to admit you're curious, because so-and-so, whose body is looking great, does it. And you don't want to admit that so-and-so's body is looking great or that you even notice how so-and-so looks in the first place.

- You know you want to try it but just haven't followed through because of some other likely and completely understandable reason.

It doesn't matter how fit, enthusiastic, or prepared you are, when it comes to trying out a new form of exercise, wimps come in all shapes, sizes, and levels of ability. Recently, I took up tennis for the first time in my life. When I first walked onto that court, every memory of a gym class gone bad went through my head. I kept telling myself, "I'm fit. I'm active. I can hit a ball." I felt awkward and stiff at first but remained focused and determined, and after a while it actually felt pretty good. It is the nature of any new thing to be slightly intimidating. And doing something new with our bodies, in front of a group of people, can be even more daunting. But, thankfully, life is full of new experiences and challenges. We crave them, which may be why you're holding this book in your hand now. Perhaps what you've heard about Pilates has piqued your interest. That is precisely what led me to Pilates: a craving, an instinct, something that told me, "This is what my body needs." So I listened to it.

Every Sunday at BodyTonic, I teach a basic Pilates Mat class that could be considered "Pilates for Wimps." The class is specially designed for people who are new to the technique (or any kind of exercise, for that matter), and it attracts

a broad spectrum of ages, fitness levels, and personalities. Curious newcomers show up, some older, some younger, and each with a unique personal fitness history—anything from a 19-year-old professional dancer to a 65-year-old political science professor who has never exercised in his life. These fresh new faces blend right in with "the groupies," a diverse bunch of devotees, 20-something to 60-something, who show up religiously and are quite happy to remain in the basic class indefinitely. Each week these regulars discover something new about their bodies and see progress—more strength, more flexibility, and better posture. They know they'll leave feeling wonderful for the rest of the day. Then there are those who get hooked on progressing in the Pilates technique, for whom the class is a prelude to more challenging levels. For them, the basic (wimp) class is just a pit stop before joining the intermediate (die-hard) class. Whatever their individual goals, all the students get something out of the class. Young, old, out of shape, in shape, Pilates is for everyone, and I'm reminded of that each time I teach.

One of the main attractions of Pilates is that it is simultaneously challenging and kind to the body. Results come free of pain or strain, with just a touch of soreness when you've hit a spot that's been pretty much dead for a while. Students work at their own level within a technique that is natural to the human form, and hence, they feel *good* afterward. Feeling stiff and sore is a hindrance, not a profit. Joe Pilates' concept of creating a smooth routine, with lots of strengthening (where every exercise works your *entire* body) and lots of stretching (where every exercise lengthens the body) is pure genius. And so much of it is done lying down! Clients have mused that they just love lying down and exercising at the same time, and that's what keeps them coming back. But my memory is loaded with the myriad other reasons why they've become addicts: They feel completely energized after class. Carrying their groceries is easier. They love their new, chiseled arms and better posture. They sleep better. They feel more relaxed. Lower back pain vanishes. Clothes fit better. Whatever the reason, when they miss a session or class, they admit they actually crave it.

The majority of us simply need to spend more time with our bodies. In the midst of a fitness boom, there are still many people who are wondering how and what they can squeeze into their already complicated schedules. But it doesn't have to be difficult, time-consuming, or unpleasant to add physical and mental conditioning to your life. *Pilates for Wimps* offers a framework for doing this with ease and intelligence. I will present the basic tools and philosophy to get you going. You will build a routine for yourself one step at a time. With each step, you'll feel better physically, mentally, and spiritually—you'll see that it doesn't have to be so hard. It can actually be *fun*!

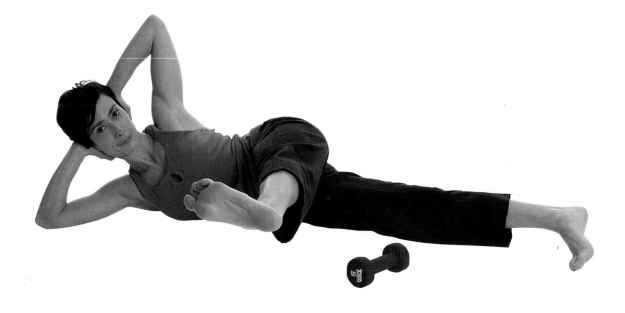

Getting Started

I truly believe people would exercise more often if they just had a menu of fun exercises tattooed on their brains. Anytime they were in need of a quick, rejuvenating body boost, they could call on a few of those strengthening and stretching moves and transform their mood from "blah" to "ahhhh. . . ." That's exactly what we're aiming for in *Pilates for Wimps*. The sections are laid out in an order designed to inspire your progress from Pilates wimp to Pilates poster child. Putting Pilates into your body little by little will have an everlasting effect—the ultimate goal is to make this method your own.

Joe Pilates was a big fan of efficiency. He knew that to get the most "bang for your buck" while you exercise, it's important to understand how to work the right muscles with the right amount of effort and the correct posture. As Joe would say, three to five well-performed repetitions of an exercise are worth a hundred sloppy repetitions. He was so right. My clients find it fuels their progress when the body is demystified. The first section in this book, "Knowledge Is Power," gives a little anatomy for wimps, so to speak. So before you dive in to the Pilates technique, take a look at the major body parts

you'll be working. I think you'll find it really helpful.

In "Instant Pilates," you'll learn—and master!—a comprehensive string of the Pilates Mat exercises. A huge part of Joe's philosophy is that the movements are performed one after the other in a continuous stream of dynamic and flowing movement. So they occur in a specific order, based on a specific level of ability. In this section, you're getting a total package of the basics for the average person. I have divided the sequence into different sections so you can learn it a bit a time or, if you have time for only a couple of exercises, you can choose a section to focus on. To see the quickest results, I recommend starting at the beginning and adding on bit by bit. It's really exciting when you're able to remember a routine and have it at your fingertips.

Joe also had a knack for how to deal with everyday complaints and general malaise, both physical and mental. "Fix-Its" provides you with a selection of handy tools for curing what ails you. You will find that, through the Pilates method of exercise, your body awareness will greatly increase. When you notice you are in need of a particular type

of soothing on a particular day—say, tight neck muscles or a depressed mood—you'll find what you need here.

Because Joe Pilates designed his technique for students to progress, I am honoring this aspect of his philosophy by including a section called "Bonus Points!" In it, you'll find more advanced versions of some of the exercises you've already learned, plus new, challenging exercises to work on when you're ready to turn things up a notch or two. Again, remember that it's all supposed to happen in a specific order, so as you move along, you should splice the new exercises into your existing routine. The "Bonus Points!" section shows you a complete, seamless more advanced version to aspire to.

Keep in mind that, as in all aspects of life, it's important to work in the appropriate amount of challenge. Biting off more than you can chew can cause an immense amount of stress. On the flip side, when you're not challenged enough, you feel bored and uninspired. Your body reacts the same way with exercise. So do what you can, do it well, and move on to the next challenge when you're ready.

Who Is Joe?

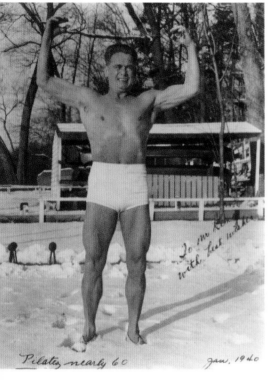

Photo courtesy of The PhysicalMind Institute

Joseph Hubertus Pilates, the mastermind behind this whole craze, was born in 1880 in a town near Dusseldorf, Germany. As a child, he struggled with a litany of physical ailments. He was a scrawny kid who suffered bouts with asthma, rickets, and rheumatic fever but was somehow fiercely determined to live a vital life. Dedicating himself to a variety of physical training methods, he became a pillar of health. He studied yoga, acrobatics, boxing, and circus arts, and his years of training in these Eastern and Western forms of exercise, combined with his unyielding desire for health, make up the foundation of what we know as Pilates.

By 1928 Joe had immigrated to New York City with his wife, Clara, and was teaching out of a studio on Eighth Avenue. He had designed several different pieces of very odd-looking equipment; devised the entire Mat routine, which he called "Contrology"; and developed a philosophy of health and fitness to go along with it all. In the early 20th century, nothing like this existed anywhere. Word spread, and the physical elite began to embrace his method. Dance legends such as Martha Graham, Hanya Holm, and George Balanchine used his method for their dance companies and often sent principal dancers to his studio for instruction.

An eccentric man who loved to throw around powerful, dramatic, and often astonishingly verbose statements about the body, Joe was promoting mind/body fitness at a time when people still considered the vibrating belt to be a viable fitness regimen. (I don't think the phrase "mind/body fitness" was used until the 1980s). In *Your Health*, a book he wrote way back in 1934, a whole chapter is entitled "The Balance of Body and Mind." In it he asserts, quite intensely, that

> ". . . neither the body or the mind is supreme—the one cannot be subordinated by the other. Both must be coordinated, in order not only to accomplish the maximum results with the minimum expenditure of mental and physical energy, but also to live as long as possible in normal health and enjoy the benefits of a useful and happy life."

Joe's writings aptly demonstrate that he was a man born with a purpose. *Your Health* was an attempt to enlighten the general population through his philosophies. He found the ignorance in the United States to be mind-boggling and at times harshly criticized doctors, parents, and the "modern business-man" for this lack of awareness. He was bothered by the excessive use of medications. He was angry with parents for expecting children to sit still when they should be active. And he was flabbergasted at the idea that people would run after wealth at the expense of the body's well being.

In 1945, Joe wrote *Return to Life Through Contrology*. It contains a solidly developed series of corrective and restorative exercises that anyone can perform at home. But the book is more than a list of exercises; it is his personal crusade to restore mental and physical health in this country, to correct the ills imposed on the human body in "this Modern Age."

Joe believed that a normal, healthy body is "your birthright!" but that only through a commitment to physical health could you hope to maintain that right. It was up to you, not a doctor, to practice simple prevention and maintenance. A few simple exercises, perfectly executed and consistently performed, would keep you in great shape mentally *and* physically, leaving you with tons of energy for work, sports, socializing, and emergencies. By now he had 20 years of experience to prove his methods and ideology. Back then, though, average Americans still wanted the dollar, the prescription, and—if they *were* exercising—the big, bulky, immobile muscles that come

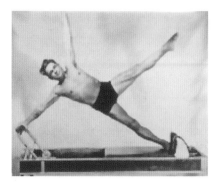

Photo courtesy of The PhysicalMind Institute

only with tiresome workouts. Joe's were exercises for *everyone*. Maintenance for the masses, whether young or old, flabby or fit! He was 60 years ahead of his time, and he knew it.

Luckily, there were those who gave Pilates a try, and many of them stuck with it. The benefits were immediate and simply too obvious to ignore. With sessions no longer than one hour (he is frequently quoted as saying "An hour . . . in the shower!"), his pupils looked toned and moved gracefully. They walked out of the studio feeling taller, stronger, more limber, and relaxed and yet energized. Their immune systems grew stronger, and postural deviations once thought unchangeable showed improvement. The same is entirely true of Pilates today with proper use of the technique, consistency, and a good teacher.

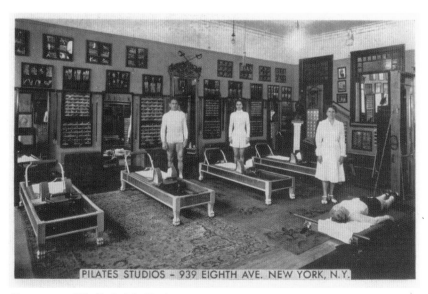

PILATES STUDIOS · 939 EIGHTH AVE. NEW YORK, N.Y.

Photo courtesy of The PhysicalMind Institute

What Is the Pilates Mat?

What Joe called Contrology is known around the world today as the Pilates Mat. Although some of the exercises have been slightly altered from their original versions based on further research and practice, the routine is the same, and the principles haven't lost their impact. You might have seen a Pilates Mat class advertised at a local fitness studio or gym, but it doesn't require any equipment other than a mat and you. It's great for your body and your mind and can be done anywhere, anytime—by anyone. In fact, that's exactly what Joe intended!

The Pilates Mat is a series of simple, fluid, and efficient exercises performed one right after the other. They alternate tension and relaxation, full expansion and contraction to give you both strength and stretch. Throughout the routine you work your entire body, focusing on your abdominal muscles whether you're using them to move or to stabilize yourself. In this way, you build a strong center while stretching and strengthening the spine, neck, arms, and legs. The various movements and body positions are specifically designed to work small muscles and large muscles in a balanced way so that all are utilized, no weaknesses persist, and nothing becomes overde-

veloped. Special attention is given to the spinal column to improve posture and lubricate and rejuvenate the cushiony, cartilaginous discs between your vertebrae. The movements, performed in different body positions and using the floor, massage your muscles and internal organs—your body not only looks better, it feels better.

At first glance, some of the exercises might not seem all that difficult, but the challenge is in their simplicity. To achieve the proper alignment and a smooth rhythm requires attention, awareness, and strength. It's like working out, meditating, going to the chiropractor, and getting a massage all in one!

THE SIX POINTS OF PILATES

Through the years, the ideology behind the madness has been boiled down to six basic principles. These are the foundation of the Pilates technique, and they explain "the work within the work." For instance, doing the Arm Series is great! But how you do your Arm Series makes all the difference between minor and major benefits. If you are looking to get the most out of every movement, consider these six points to be your stepping-stones.

Concentration

This is one of the most valuable principles of the technique (and one of my personal favorites), because the power of concentration enables you to learn so much about your body. Complete concentration also truly relaxes you. Bringing your mind and your body together for just 10 minutes without distraction will have a lasting, positive effect on your soul for the rest of the day. And, to put it bluntly, if you wish to profit from the other five principles, you'll need to focus. Some Pilates Mat exercises are simply impossible to do if you're thinking about something else.

Control

This might be where Joe's German upbringing and the American psychology of the Depression era come into play, but you won't find any wasted movement in Pilates. Ironically, performing the movements with complete control—no wasted movement—improves your ability to "fling about" later. Take tennis, skiing, or running after your kids: These activities all require quick reactions and weight shifts, things that, without proper control, might leave you flat on your face. After training in Pilates, your body has been programmed

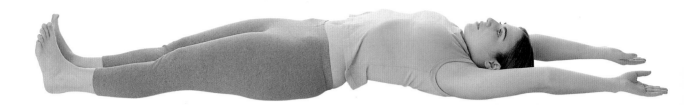

to move efficiently, in a way that's balanced and stable, but limber. That coordination becomes deeply ingrained in your neuromuscular pathways. Bring that training to the court, the slope, or your backyard, and you won't even have to think about how to move. It will all be automatic.

Centering

Throughout the Pilates Mat, you focus on what Joe called "the powerhouse." This is the area between your rib cage and pelvis. Think of it as a corset of muscle that you are always pulling in toward an imaginary core within the body. Every movement incorporates the use of the abdominal and lower back muscles that make up this corset. Many of the Mat exercises are obviously focused on working your abdominals, but even the ones that seem like just arm or leg exercises challenge the powerhouse. Its central support provides the stability necessary to allow the rest of your body to move freely. As your limbs move, this weave of muscles acting on your torso prevents you from losing control. There are also the cosmetic benefits to consider: Keep pulling your abdominals in toward your center, and your efforts will translate into a shrinking waistline. Nice!

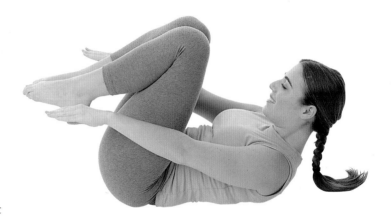

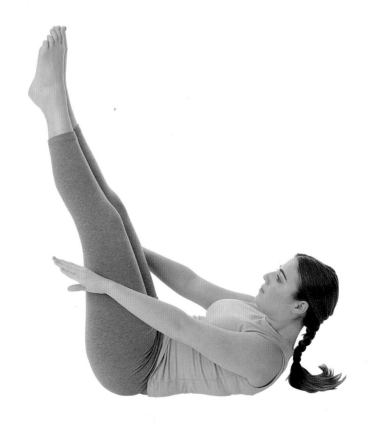

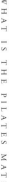

Deep Breathing

While doing the Pilates Mat routine, take full, deep, luscious breaths; when you exhale, try to push all the air out of your lungs. In the beginning this may leave you a little light-headed, but as you practice, your body will become accustomed to the higher level of oxygen. Every movement in the Pilates Mat is coordinated with an inhalation and an exhalation. Generally, you inhale in expanded positions and exhale in contracted ones. Coordinating breath and movement this way sharpens your focus, enhances your rhythm, helps you move with greater ease, and synchronizes your mind, muscles, and respiratory system. The increased oxygen flow to the brain revives you like a cup of coffee, and getting more oxygen to the muscles gives them power, stamina, and flexibility. Deep breathing also helps rid the body of toxins and debris in the lungs, so you'll breathe better even when you're not exercising.

Precision

Joe felt that one movement performed five times perfectly was worth hours of sloppy exertion. To get the true value out of an exercise, it must be done properly. Otherwise, you're practicing a bad habit, and as with any bad habit, your body will pay you back in time. This precision might take extra effort at first, but it gets really exciting as you progress. Your body becomes a fine-tuned instrument, mastering all your movements, whether you're exercising or doing everyday activities. You might think that precision is an annoying, nit-picky kind of quality, but I find that the opposite is true. People really enjoy doing something correctly. And they immediately feel the benefits of moving with proper alignment and efficient muscular effort.

Flowing Movement

One of the most attractive qualities of the Pilates Mat is that it was designed to be a continuous stream of movement. That flow inspires grace, encourages economy of movement, soothes the body, and adds an aerobic component to the technique. Most people think exercise has to be uncomfortable, monotonous, and jarring to be cardiovascular, but it really boils down to moving without stopping. In Pilates you move continuously in a way that's kind to the body—smoothly, gracefully, fluidly, efficiently. Care has been taken to provide transitions that shift you seamlessly from one position to the next. I think a lot of people enjoy the concept of entering into this rhythmic continuum as they start their Mat routine. It has a truly meditative effect, like that of a beautiful song or a flawless dance. When you're finished, your mental and physical faculties feel balanced and soothed, responsive yet relaxed.

The beauty of these basic principles lies in the way they work together. Deep breathing helps you to concentrate. Concentrating helps you to center. Centering helps you to control your movements, and so on. These elemental combinations give birth to great rewards. They unite the body and mind, help you to execute your movements with ease, and keep you in control of the motion instead of letting the motion control you. The exercises you practice will move quickly into the subconscious, and when that happens, you "own" the work. It belongs to you, not an instructor or an apparatus. Now you can do your Pilates Mat routine and reap its benefits anytime, anywhere—and on your own.

Last-Minute Tips

Before we start moving, here are some important items and ideas to help you in your Pilates practice.

A FEW PROPS YOU WILL NEED

- A small area of wall with no obstructions.

- Two neckties or bathrobe belts.

- Carpeting, a mat, or a couple of towels to cushion you when lying on the floor.

- Two thick blankets or pillows.

- Two soup cans or light weights (one, two, or five pounds each).

- A chair.

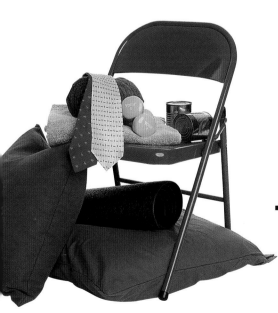

FINAL WORDS TO GET YOU GOING

- Remember to breathe—and do so from your rib cage, because when you're busy pulling your belly button in and up, it's difficult to breathe into your abdomen. Concentrate on expanding your ribs instead.

- If you feel any kind of pain, stop! Your body is telling you the exercise doesn't work for you. Come back to it another day or have the pain checked out by a specialist.

- Wear loose, comfortable clothing and no shoes. Socks are fine, but you don't need them.

- Joe designed the technique so one movement would flow into the next, so learn the exercises in order. My advice would be to add an exercise or a section each time you practice. Eventually you'll be able to zip through the entire routine in 20 minutes. Really! It's a great thing to pull out of your pocket after a road trip, airline flight, or long workday.

- If you don't have time for the entire Pilates Mat sequence, just do a section. I recommend doing even a little bit every other day.

- Try to let all unnecessary tension in other areas of your body drain into your powerhouse. For instance, if your neck and shoulders are tight, imagine sucking that tension into your abdominals.

- Shoulder hunching is a universal problem. Think of your shoulder blades sliding down into your back pockets throughout your practice.

- If one side of your body is weaker than the other, do a few extra moves on the weaker side to help strengthen those muscles.

- Be consistent with your practice. To stay motivated, do it with a friend, take a class, change your schedule—whatever you have to do. The body loves consistency, and you'll feel greater rewards if you stick with it.

- When you have the opportunity, study with a competent teacher. It's helpful to have a pair of skilled eyes watch and guide you.

- Have fun!

Knowledge Is Power

Ever feel like a complete clutz in a class? Or wonder why the instructor has abdominal muscles while you were somehow born without them? You're not alone—I hear these concerns all the time. But I have discovered that there's a graceful mover with a complete set of working abdominals in everyone. As a Pilates neophyte, increasing your knowledge of the body will be a springboard to new levels of achievement, including fluid movement and a firm midsection. Fortunately, I'm a total anatomy geek—nothing excites me more than demystifying the body for those of you who would rather not bury your face in a medical textbook. And I love drumming up clear, simple (and sometimes bizarre) imagery to demonstrate anatomy and simplify the technical aspects of proper alignment. A blanket understanding of the body's architecture is all you need to greatly increase the benefits of the time you spend exercising or doing everyday activities. As a matter of fact, even if you aren't up for exercising, a glance at this section will inspire you to maintain an elegant posture for the remainder of the day. On some days that might be the only workout you need!

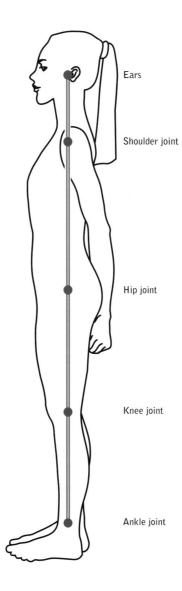

Ears

Shoulder joint

Hip joint

Knee joint

Ankle joint

Figure 1

VISUALIZE YOUR CENTRAL AXIS

The body is an architecturally sound structure. All your parts can be balanced around a vertical axis—imagine a broomstick running though the center of your body from head to foot. Ideally, ears, shoulders, hips, knees, and ankles should be arranged symmetrically on either side of this axis, and although your natural curves differ from front to back, they should be balanced on either side of this central line. If the body is off balance, some muscle somewhere will have to work overtime, becoming strained and overdeveloped, which in turn means another muscle gets to slack off, eventually resulting in a debilitating weakness. Your alignment "checkpoints"—ankles, knees, hips, shoulders, and ears—are noted from the side view in Figure 1. To encourage skeletal and muscular balance, visualize your axis as you do your Mat work by moving through and rotating around this central line. For instance, in the Roll-Up (see page TK), you are rolling and unrolling through your central line. In the Saw (see page TK), when you twist, you are spiraling around your central axis.

LENGTHEN ALONG AND HUG THE AXIS

Once all your parts are balanced, think of stretching out along the axis. When standing, you should feel as if the very top of your head is piercing the ceiling—imagine that you're wearing a really dorky party hat with its pointy tip aimed directly upward. At the same time, your feet are pressing the floor away. When you're lying down, imagine that you're on the rack, your party hat stretching toward the wall behind you while your tailbone, legs, and feet stretch the opposite direction. Imagine your alignment checkpoints moving away from your belly button. Next, think of all of the muscles in your midsection, or powerhouse, hugging the axis. It's sort of like sucking in when you're trying on a tight pair of jeans. In essence, the energy is pulling in 360 degrees around your waist, then shooting out through the top of your head, through your legs, through the tips of your fingers. It's like you have this fireball of energy in your midsection, and the rest of your body radiates outward from that. (A lot of people use the image of a sun and its rays while doing Mat work.) All that stuff you've heard about Pilates building long, lean muscle and a strong midsection comes from focusing on this aspect of the technique. So, suck in and s-t-r-e-t-c-h out for all your exercises!

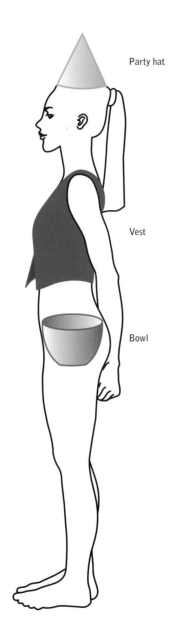

Party hat

Vest

Bowl

Figure 2

STACK THE BOWL, THE VEST, AND THE PARTY HAT
(See Figure 2.)

Inspiring people to stand or sit properly can be a tricky thing. If I bark commands like "Stand up straight!" or "Sit tall!" I get people sticking their chests out and poking their chins in the air—and no one's breathing! So instead I talk people through balancing the pelvis, rib cage, and skull. Let's begin with the center of life itself, the **pelvis**. The word *pelvis* means "basin" in Latin, and that is the perfect image for this bowl-shaped bony structure.

When standing or sitting, the bottom of your pelvic bowl should face the floor, and the top should face the rib cage. This is important because the pelvis carries the weight of your internal organs, spine, upper limbs, brain, head . . . everything up there! If it's angled the wrong way, something above will have to tip the opposite way to compensate; and something below—your knee, for example—will have too much weight to bear. Now, the **rib cage**: The shape of your rib cage is much like a cropped vest, and the bottom of it should hover directly over the pelvic bowl. To complete your elegant posture, balance the **skull** or your imaginary "party hat" above your eyes focused straight out in front of you. (Maintaining a line of sight that is parallel to the floor is a great tool for centering your skull.) Whether you're standing or sitting, that pointy top stretches up to the ceiling while the bottom of the hat hovers above the rib cage, which, of course, hovers above the pelvic bowl—three, big, bony structures completely in alignment. This is important because when they are off balance, it can wreak havoc on the muscles straining to keep things together.

ANATOMY OF THE POWERHOUSE—FRONT TO BACK
(See Figure 3.)

The space between the rib cage and the pelvis is where the internal organs work their magic. The only bones in this area are five little lumbar vertebrae, so it's up to the powerhouse to maintain the integrity and strength of the torso. The powerhouse is an intense support network made up of a complex weave of abdominal and spinal muscles, with fibers running horizontally, vertically, and diagonally to reinforce the connection of the rib cage to the pelvis. Here's a brief breakdown:

Transversus abdominis: A broad, flat muscle with fibers that run horizontally, covering the area from your pubic bone to about your lower six ribs. It connects to the rectus abdominis in front and the erector spinae in back. This is your "suck-in-your-gut" muscle.

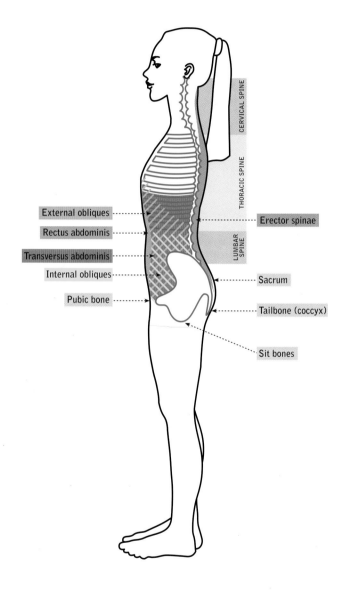

External obliques
Rectus abdominis
Transversus abdominis
Internal obliques
Pubic bone

CERVICAL SPINE
THORACIC SPINE
LUMBAR SPINE

Erector spinae
Sacrum
Tailbone (coccyx)
Sit bones

Figure 3

Rectus abdominis: The long, flat pair of muscles that run vertically along the front of your body from the pubic bone to about the fifth rib (one muscle is on the left, and the other is on the right). These are your "six-pack" abs, and you use them to flex the spine forward (see the Hundred, page TK).

Internal and external oblique abdominals: Two different layers of muscle with fibers that slant in opposite directions to reinforce the sides of your body. They run from the top of the pelvis and pubic bone to about the fifth rib and to the pectoral muscles. They are used when you bend sideways or twist, and they help you complete a full Roll-Up (see page TK).

Erector spinae: A group of muscles with fibers that run vertically along the back of your body from pelvis to skull. These muscles work to extend the spine backward (see the Swimming, page TK), allow us to bend side to side, help us to stand up when we're bent over, and twist the torso.

Basically, the four types of abdominal muscles support your body in the front, maintain pressure on the lower back to protect it, and contract to flex you forward. Your erector spinae muscles support the spine in back and work to extend the spine backward. Both sets of oblique muscles support the sides of your body and help to accomplish the tasks of twisting and side bending. And all these muscles work as stabilizers when you move your limbs.

Note for the Curious: For our purposes, we don't need to go much further into anatomy, but here's a little additional information, if you want it, regarding the limbs. Your arms connect to your midsection mainly through the **latissimmus dorsi**, the big fan-like muscles that run from the shoulder joints to the middle spine and down the sides of your body, weaving into your **obliques**. Your legs are connected via your **psoas** muscles, which run from your lower back to the femur, or thighbone. I could go on and on here, so if you're still curious, check out your local bookstore for an anatomy book that appeals to you.

A WORD ABOUT THE SPINE

Some people might feel like their spine is just one stiff pole, but it is wonderfully designed to accommodate a full range of movements. Your **vertebral column**, or spine, has twenty four vertebrae of varying sizes, with cushiony discs in between. This design functions magnificently to absorb shock as your feet hit the ground, whether strolling through the park or playing a game of one-on-one. It allows you to bend forward, backward, and sideways, as well as to twist, and it helps support the weight of the upper body. At the base of the spine is the **coccyx**, or tailbone, which is the bottom tip of the centerpiece of your pelvis: a triangular bone called the **sacrum**. Your spine extends upward from the sacrum to the skull, where it attaches right in the back, between your ears. Five **lumbar vertebrae** support the

lower back, twelve **thoracic vertebrae** support the ribs, and seven **cervical vertebrae** support the neck and head (which weighs roughly 8 pounds). Between each pair of vertebrae is a cushiony **intervertebral disc**. Ligaments act as cables, attaching vertebra to vertebra and helping keep it all in place. Aside from being structurally responsible for the wide-ranging motion of your torso and the support of your upper body, the spine encases and protects the **spinal cord** and **nerve roots** that make up your central nervous system. Keep in mind, those shock-absorbing intervertebral discs have been under pressure since the day you first sat up. With aging, they are going to dehydrate and thin—and with a chronic misalignment, your chances of developing a bulging or herniated disc can be quite high. Properly aligned stretching and strengthening can offset this. Joseph Pilates often proclaimed that the secret to staying young was keeping the spine stretched, strong, and supple. So as you move, focus on your posture and think about creating space between the vertebrae to allow your intervertebral discs to expand and rejuvenate!

Note: Abnormal curvature of the spine—such as scoliosis, lordosis, and kyphosis—is quite common. Consistent, well-performed Pilates practice can help to minimize these conditions.

As you stand at the threshold of an exciting and new physical life, consider this oft-quoted piece of wisdom from Joseph Pilates' himself: "It is the mind which governs the body." Joe believed that your Pilates practice (or any exercise, for that matter) should fully utilize what are widely believed to be the five parts of the mind— will, intuition, intelligence, imagination, and memory. Repeat Joe's phrase to yourself right now, and carry these thoughts with you every time you practice. Make the phrase your own personal exercise mantra. Along with the visual and written information on the pages ahead, this concept is all you need for an exceptional fitness experience. Get ready to achieve new feats of athleticism with grace and ease. Let your mind be your guide and you'll discover the pace that's exactly right for you.

1

Instant Pilates *The Exercises*

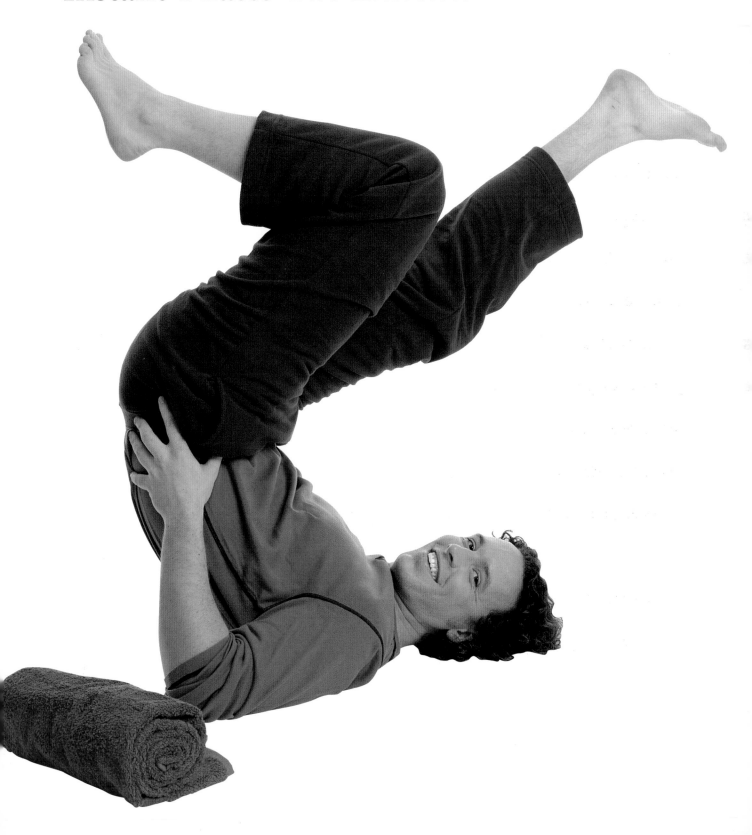

Start Me Up!

Here we go. The next four exercises will get your heart pumping, blood circulating, and oxygen flowing. We're going to fire up your abs and warm up your legs and spine. Remember, this is a time to bring your mind and body together. If you need to lie down and take a few deep breaths to center yourself before you begin, please do so. I sometimes tell my students to imagine they're a bottle of fizzy soda. Open the bottle and let any nagging thoughts float out the top of your head like bubbles. It's also a great idea to unplug the phone!

Starting position for the Mat routine: Be sure you have enough room to completely stretch your arms above your head and your legs along the floor. You should be able to make "snow angels" without knocking into anything. Spread out your mat or towel and lie down with your tailbone and head on it. Have any accessories you might need—pillows, straps, blankets, small weights—nearby.

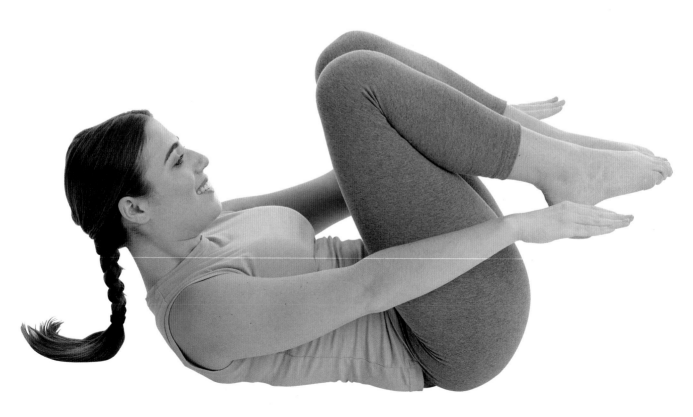

THE HUNDRED

- Lie on your back, bring your knees in to your chest, and stretch your legs toward the ceiling as straight as possible. Pull your stomach in and lift your head, shoulders, and arms off the floor.

- Pump your arms at your sides at a brisk tempo, breathing in for 5 pumps and exhaling for 5. Think of pressing the air down toward the floor with each pump. Keep your body completely still as your arms stimulate oxygen and blood flow.

- Do this for 10 deep breaths. That's 10 pumps times 10 breaths—a total of 100 counts, which is why it's called the Hundred.

- Don't worry if you can't do 100 at first. Get as close as you can, taking a rest if you have to, then add a few more next time.

TIP! If you feel strain on your back or neck, bend your knees. If you need to modify a little more, keep going with the pumps but rest your head on the floor.

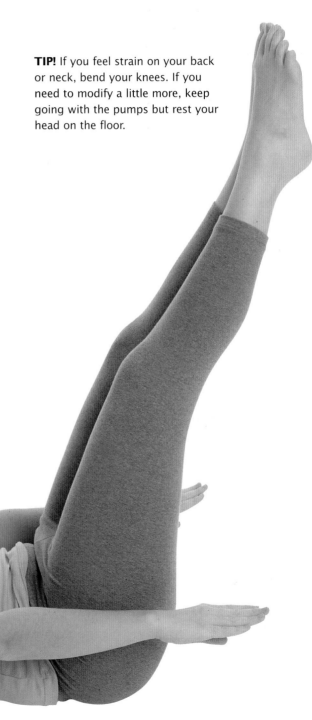

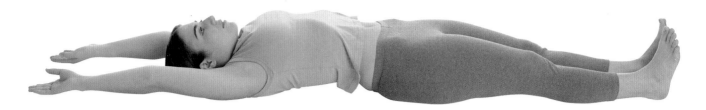

Transition: Lower your feet, head, and shoulders to the floor, then stretch your arms overhead and your legs out straight, keeping them together.

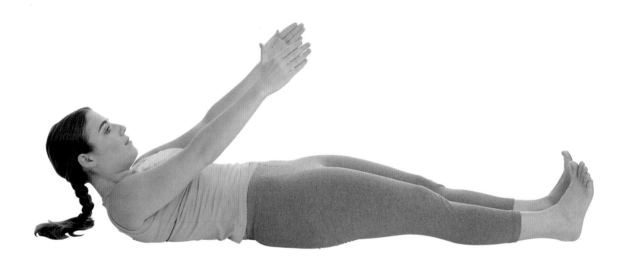

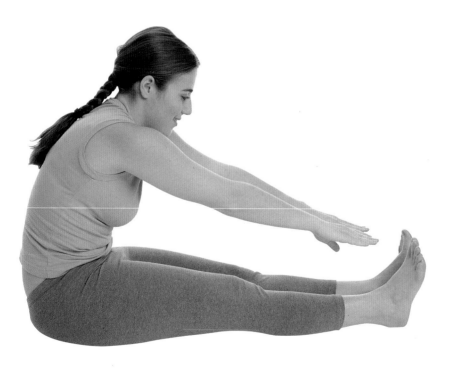

THE ROLL-UP

- Slowly bring your arms up toward the ceiling, then peel your head, shoulders, and spine off the floor bone by bone until you are stretching over your legs.

- Inhale as your head and shoulders come off the floor; exhale as you stretch over your legs. Then inhale as you start to roll back and exhale to complete the roll down. Try to make an imprint with one vertebra at a time.

- Repeat 5 times.

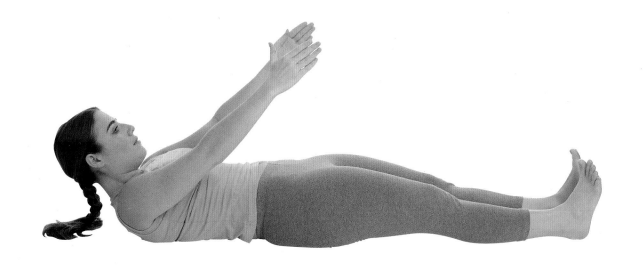

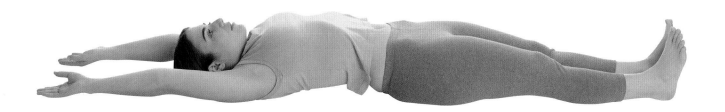

TIP! A lot of people get "stuck" at a certain point—usually when the hip flexors and rectus abdominis muscles stop doing most of the work and the oblique abdominals kick in.

Most people's obliques just aren't strong enough at first. If this happens, bend your knees and grab on to your legs to help you get up with the proper form.

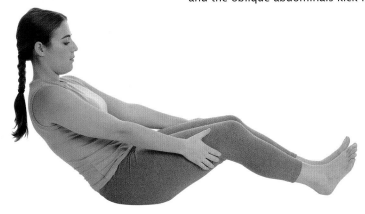

Transition: Relax back onto the floor and bring your arms down to your sides.

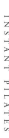

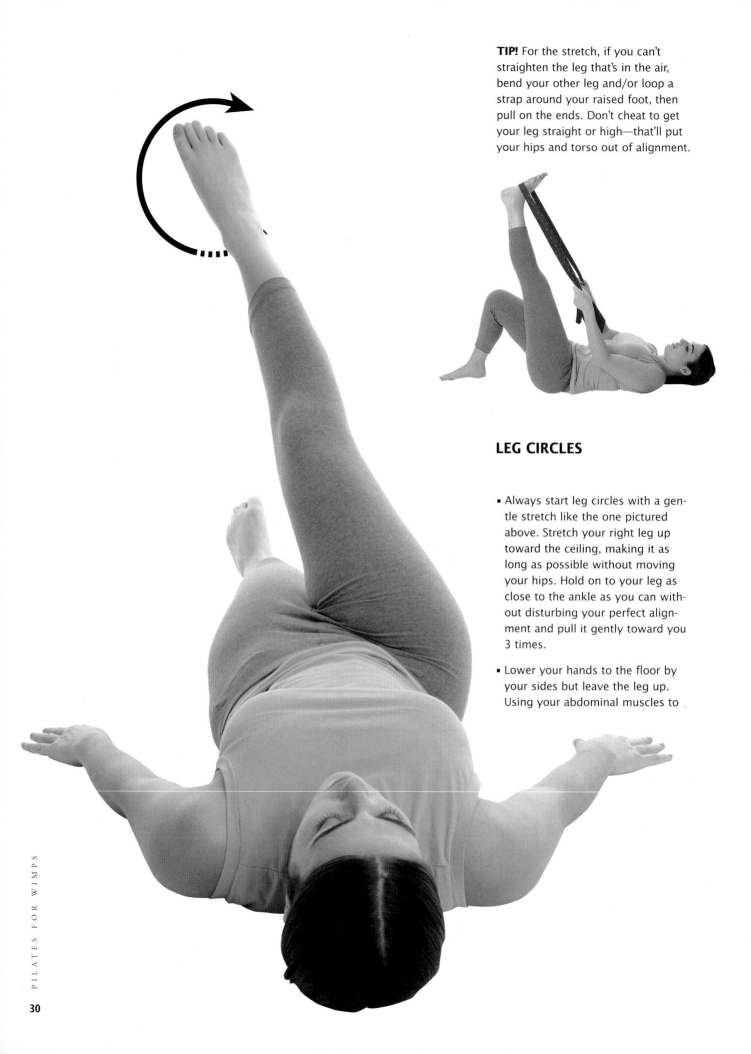

TIP! For the stretch, if you can't straighten the leg that's in the air, bend your other leg and/or loop a strap around your raised foot, then pull on the ends. Don't cheat to get your leg straight or high—that'll put your hips and torso out of alignment.

LEG CIRCLES

- Always start leg circles with a gentle stretch like the one pictured above. Stretch your right leg up toward the ceiling, making it as long as possible without moving your hips. Hold on to your leg as close to the ankle as you can without disturbing your perfect alignment and pull it gently toward you 3 times.

- Lower your hands to the floor by your sides but leave the leg up. Using your abdominal muscles to

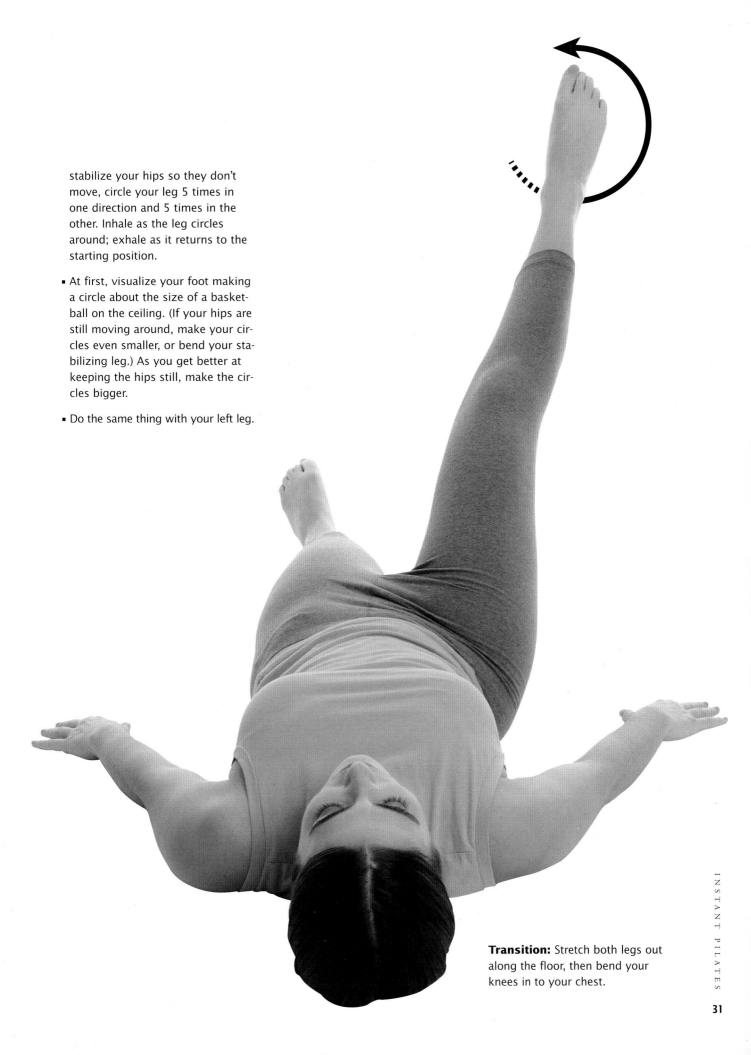

stabilize your hips so they don't
move, circle your leg 5 times in
one direction and 5 times in the
other. Inhale as the leg circles
around; exhale as it returns to the
starting position.

- At first, visualize your foot making
  a circle about the size of a basketball on the ceiling. (If your hips are
  still moving around, make your circles even smaller, or bend your stabilizing leg.) As you get better at
  keeping the hips still, make the circles bigger.

- Do the same thing with your left leg.

Transition: Stretch both legs out
along the floor, then bend your
knees in to your chest.

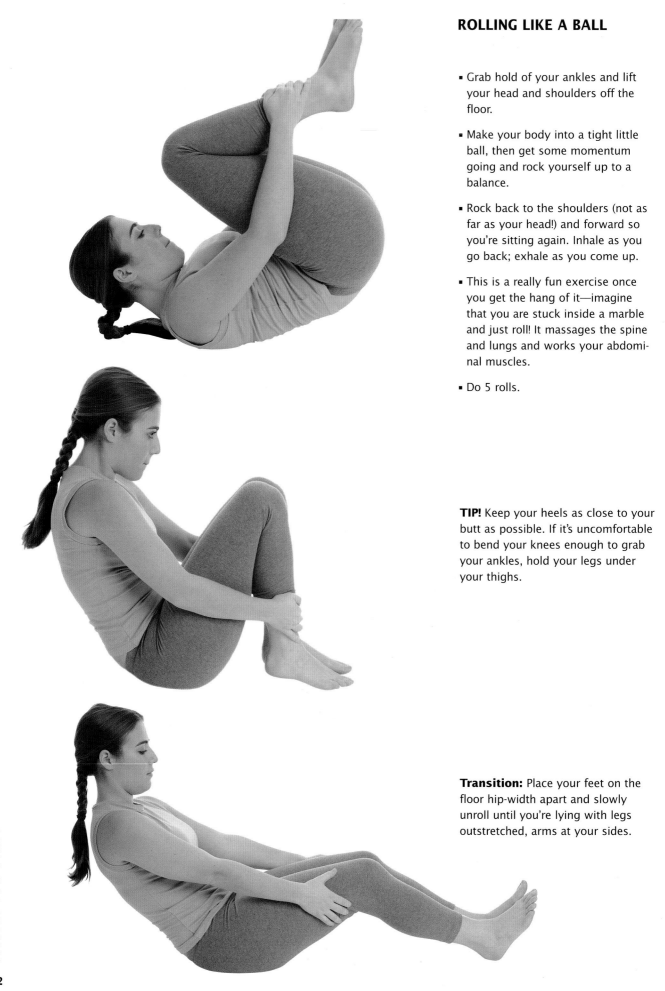

ROLLING LIKE A BALL

- Grab hold of your ankles and lift your head and shoulders off the floor.

- Make your body into a tight little ball, then get some momentum going and rock yourself up to a balance.

- Rock back to the shoulders (not as far as your head!) and forward so you're sitting again. Inhale as you go back; exhale as you come up.

- This is a really fun exercise once you get the hang of it—imagine that you are stuck inside a marble and just roll! It massages the spine and lungs and works your abdominal muscles.

- Do 5 rolls.

TIP! Keep your heels as close to your butt as possible. If it's uncomfortable to bend your knees enough to grab your ankles, hold your legs under your thighs.

Transition: Place your feet on the floor hip-width apart and slowly unroll until you're lying with legs outstretched, arms at your sides.

The Stomach Series

In this section, as your legs and arms perform different motions, your powerhouse is working hard to stabilize your torso and keep it completely still. The ultimate goal—and it's quite challenging—is to get through all the exercises one right after the other, without lowering your head and shoulders. Use your belly button as a visual aide, both to remind yourself to keep "sucking in" and to mark the center of your body. If your neck starts to get tired or you feel unnecessary strain in your back, your abs have probably had enough. Take a break. Relax back onto the floor, then think of using your abdominals to pick your head and shoulders up again.

You'll see some tips included below, but three things you can generally do to make things gentler are (1) raise the level of the extended leg, (2) bend your knees a little, and (3) rest your head on the floor if your neck gets tired. You will grow stronger in time. Trust me!

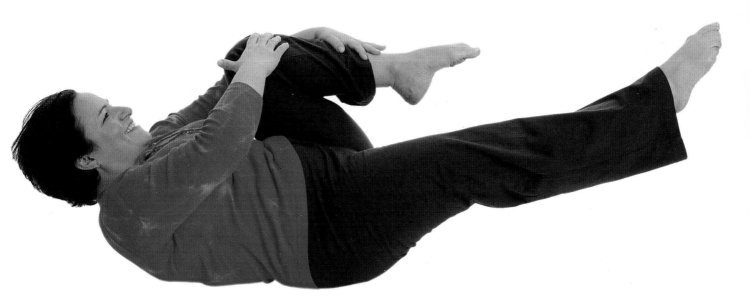

SINGLE LEG STRETCH

- Lying on your back, pull your stomach in, lift your head and shoulders off the floor, and bring your right knee up to your chest. Extend your left leg at a 45-degree angle, making sure it's in line with your belly button.

- Hold on to your bent right leg by placing your left hand on the knee and your right hand on the ankle; then pull the leg in to your chest.

- Press your stomach in, in, in! Imagine your abdomen as a body of water that keeps lowering in level.

- Change legs—and keep that water level sinking. Inhale as you pull your right leg to your chest; exhale as you pull the left.

- Do 10 stretches (5 times on each side).

DOUBLE LEG STRETCH

- Keeping your head and shoulders lifted, reach your arms overhead and stretch out both legs to a 45-degree angle, squeezing them together to work those inner thighs.

- Pull yourself into a little ball and hug your knees, then stretch your arms and legs back out. Suck in your belly extra hard in the stretched position—that's the most strenuous part.

- Inhale as you lengthen; exhale as you curl into the ball.

- Do 5 stretches.

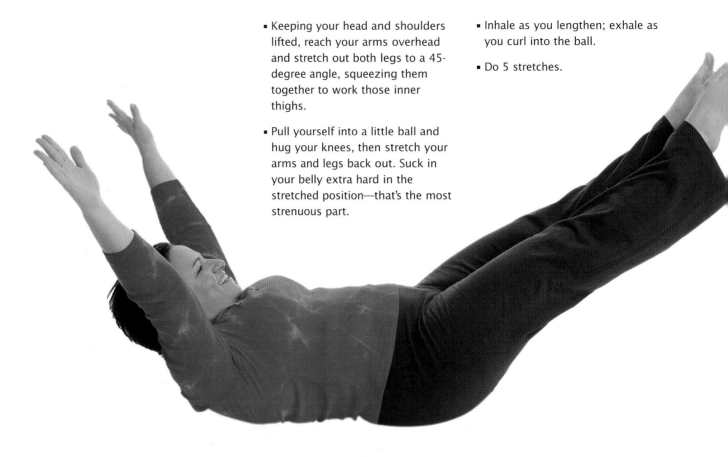

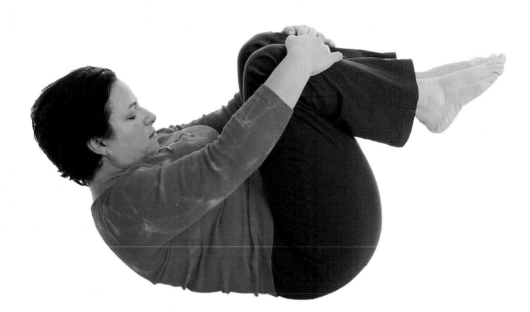

TIP! To make it easier, stretch your arms and legs toward the ceiling.

SINGLE STRAIGHT-LEG STRETCH

- Still keeping your head and shoulders off the ground, reach your right leg up straight and grab it as close to your ankle as you can. Extend your left leg at a 45-degree angle (or stretch it higher to make it easier; lower to make it harder).

- Pull the right leg toward you, using the muscles in your arms to get in some arm work along with the leg stretch.

- Switch to the left leg. Inhale while pulling the right leg; exhale while pulling the left.

- Try to keep your legs as long and stretched as possible while pulling the navel in and up. Your legs should "scissor" past one another so you know you're keeping your alignment. It's okay to take a break if you need to, but if you can do it, your head and shoulders should still be off the floor!

- Do 10 stretches (5 on each side).

TIP! If your hamstrings are super-tight, slightly bend the knee of the leg you are pulling. Eventually you'll be able to straighten it.

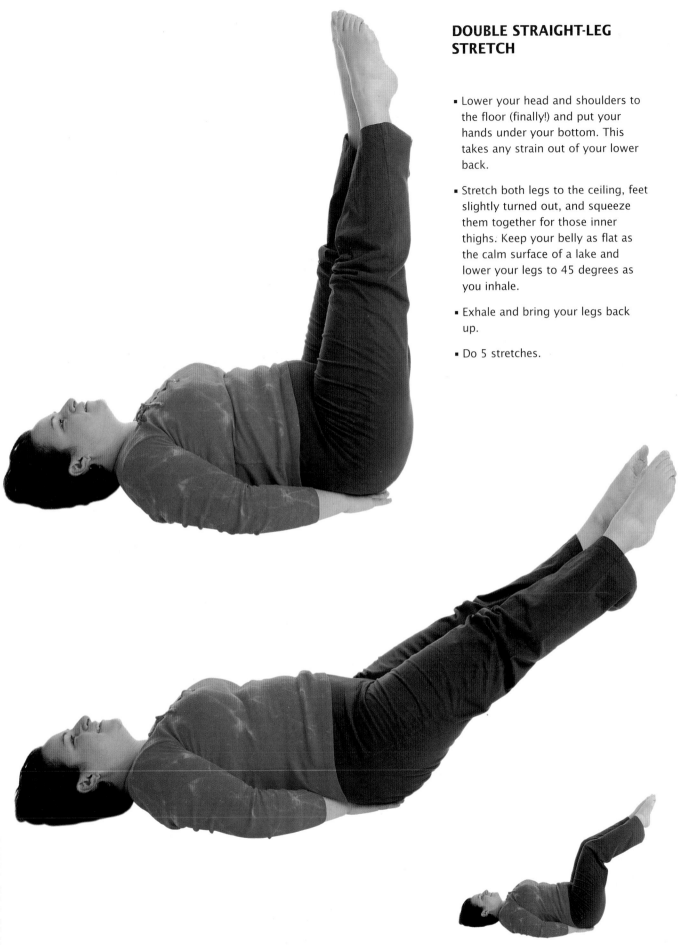

DOUBLE STRAIGHT-LEG STRETCH

- Lower your head and shoulders to the floor (finally!) and put your hands under your bottom. This takes any strain out of your lower back.

- Stretch both legs to the ceiling, feet slightly turned out, and squeeze them together for those inner thighs. Keep your belly as flat as the calm surface of a lake and lower your legs to 45 degrees as you inhale.

- Exhale and bring your legs back up.

- Do 5 stretches.

TIP! Do this with your knees bent if you feel any strain.

CRISS-CROSS

- Place your hands behind your head and lift your head and shoulders off the floor. Stretch your left leg to 45 degrees and bend your right knee into the chest.

- Without moving your pelvis (at all!), twist to touch your left elbow to your right knee. Change to do the other side. Inhale in one direction; exhale in the other.

- It's common to be able to twist more in one direction than the other. Keep an eye on this and work a little harder on your weaker side.

- Do 10 Criss-Crosses (alternating sides).

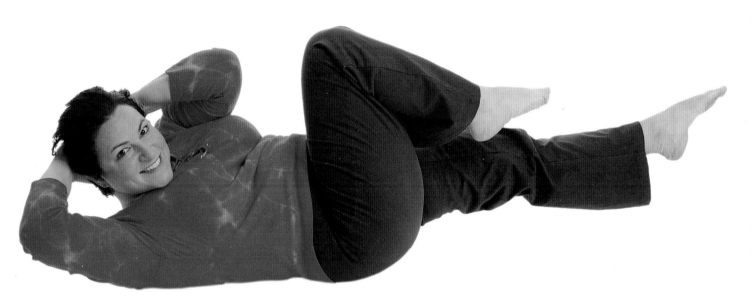

TIP! To make this easier, keep both knees bent in to the chest the entire time and just practice the upper-body part.

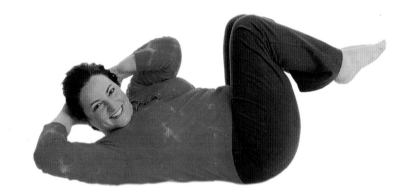

Transition: Bend both knees in to your chest (take a breath or two here, if you like) and rock up to sitting, much as in Rolling Like a Ball (see page TK).

Congratulations! You've done the Stomach Series.

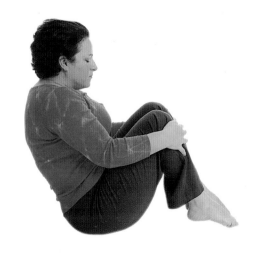

Say Hello to Your Back

The next series involves the erector spinae, the muscles that extend the spine and maintain an erect posture. In the upright sitting positions, 99 percent of my students hike their shoulders up. This doesn't surprise me; we don't spend a lot of time extending the spine. We slouch at work, lie down to watch TV, and organize our lives so that we bend down for things way more often than we reach up. Since we're stuck with these weak back muscles, our bodies struggle to sit tall—and hiking the shoulders makes us feel as if we're lifting up taller. So think of your shoulder blades sliding down your back like warm butter and take support and strength from your abdominal muscles, erector spinae, and spinal column. Remember to keep the bottom of your pelvic bowl (see page TK) directly facing the floor and the top facing the ceiling to give yourself the proper foundation. Use pillows or blankets when you need to, but if you can perform these exercises without them, great!

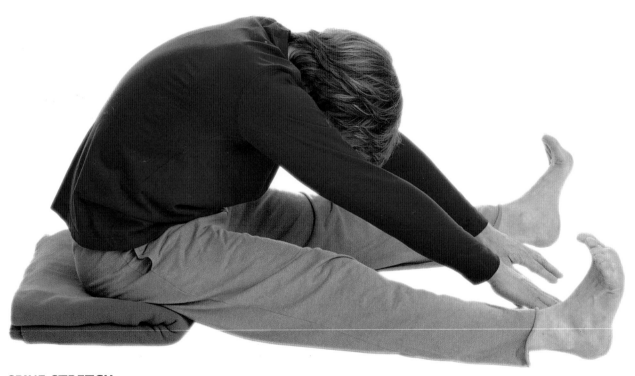

SPINE STRETCH

- From the sitting position, stretch both legs into a V. Imagine that your head has a marionette string attached to it, tugging the crown toward the sky.

- Place your fingertips in front of you on the floor (remember to keep your shoulders relaxed). Pull your tummy toward the back of the room, round your spine, reach your fingers along the floor, and stretch out through your heels. It should feel like 3 people are playing tug-of-war with your body, one grabbing your hands, one grabbing your waist, and one pulling at your heels.

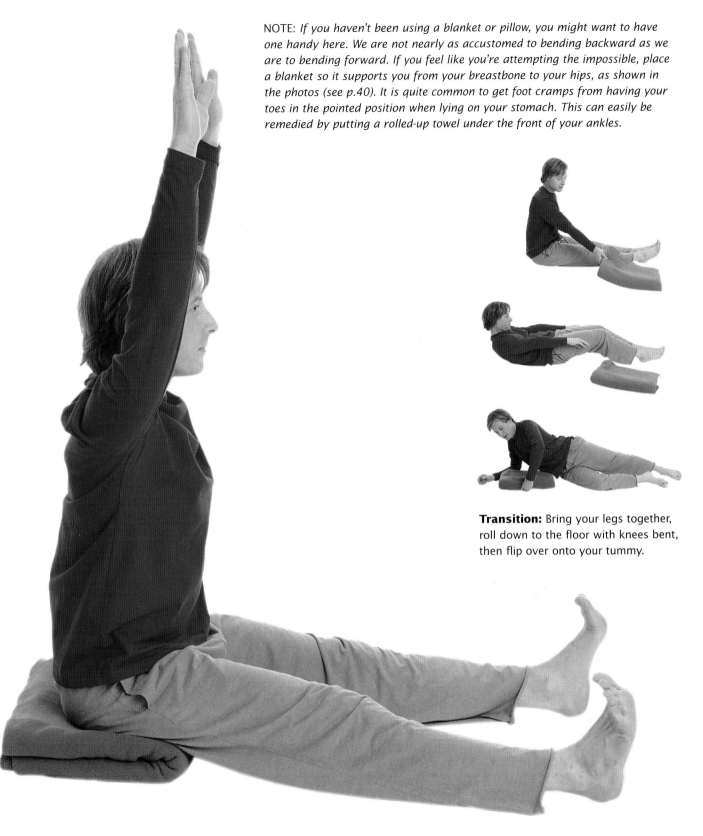

NOTE: *If you haven't been using a blanket or pillow, you might want to have one handy here. We are not nearly as accustomed to bending backward as we are to bending forward. If you feel like you're attempting the impossible, place a blanket so it supports you from your breastbone to your hips, as shown in the photos (see p.40). It is quite common to get foot cramps from having your toes in the pointed position when lying on your stomach. This can easily be remedied by putting a rolled-up towel under the front of your ankles.*

Transition: Bring your legs together, roll down to the floor with knees bent, then flip over onto your tummy.

- Exhale as you stretch your spine fully; inhale as you unroll to the sitting position by pressing the pelvis into the floor then stacking the bones of the spine one on top of

the other until your head comes up. Raise your arms to the sky.

- Do 5 stretches.

TIP! Reach your arms only as far up as your flexibility will allow. If your ribs start to stick out, you've gone too far. Your stretch will increase with practice.

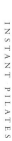

SIMPLE BACK EXTENSION

- Lie with your forehead facing the floor, legs parted slightly, and hands directly under your shoulders. Pretend there's a thumbtack sitting pointy-side up under your belly button and pull your navel up to your spine to keep a safe distance from it.

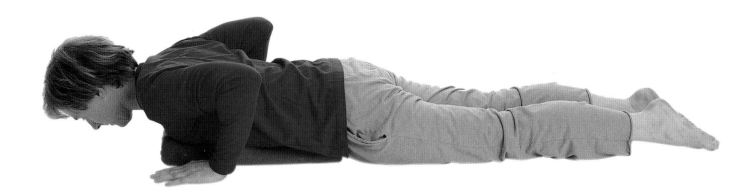

- Inhale, pushing your arms into the floor to arch up. Exhale as you lower back down to the floor.

- To keep the spine long and shoulders down, imagine that you're a turtle coming out of its shell or that you have really long earrings on and you don't want them to tickle your shoulders.

- Do 3 extensions.

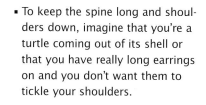

TIP! Your elbows should be pointing back, not out to the sides. This will hold your shoulders in place, work the proper arm muscles, and keep your wrists in alignment.

SINGLE LEG KICK

- Place your elbows directly under your shoulders, aim your forearms and hands straight in front of you, and bring your legs together. There's a lot going on in this starting position alone. Concentrate on pulling your belly up, pushing your arms down, and gluing your knees together. Your entire body is working!

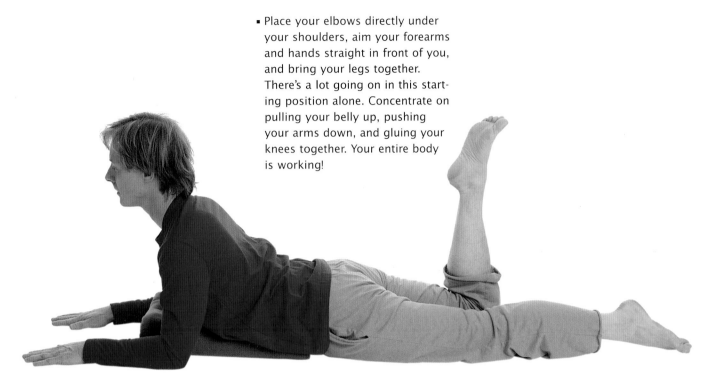

- Pulse your right foot toward your butt twice, then the left. Think of squeezing the air between your foot and your butt. Try to keep your knees together. You should feel the back of your leg working and the front of your leg stretching.

- Inhale while pulsing one leg; exhale on the other.

- Do 20 kicks (10 on each side).

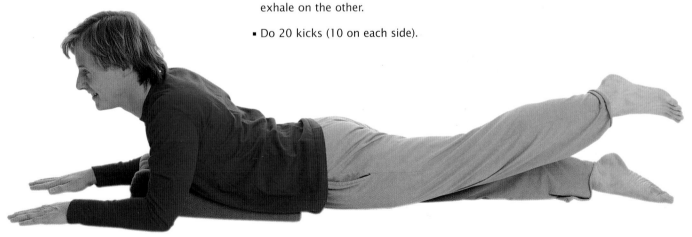

TIP! If the pulsing feels funky on your knee, leave it out or try lifting the leg straight off the floor instead. If your head is wobbling around like a bobble-head doll, you're not using the strength in your arms enough. Press harder!

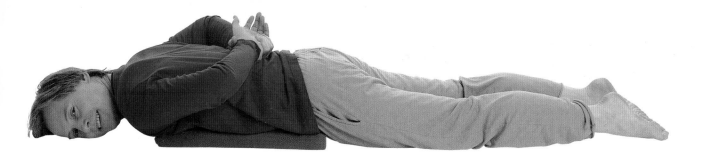

DOUBLE LEG KICK

- Lower your upper body to the floor, turning your head to the left, and grab one wrist behind your back.

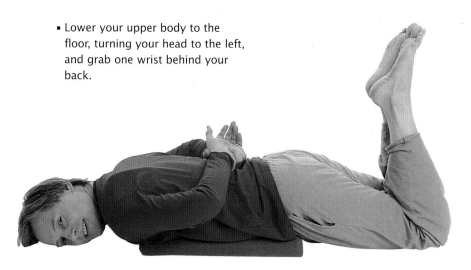

- With your knees still glued together and your tummy pulled in and up, pulse both feet toward your bottom 3 times. Return your feet to the floor and reach your arms toward your heels as you lift your chest off the floor and look straight ahead of you. Hold this for 3 counts, then lower your chest to the floor, this time turning your head to the right. So—pulse feet 1-2-3, then lift and hold 1-2-3.

- Exhale with the pulses; inhale with the lift. Try to keep your pubic bone in contact with the floor the entire time.

- Do 4 kicks.

TIP! Even if you don't come very high off the floor, try to really open your chest. Imagine that you have a flashlight attached to your breastbone and you want to shine its light on the wall in front of you.

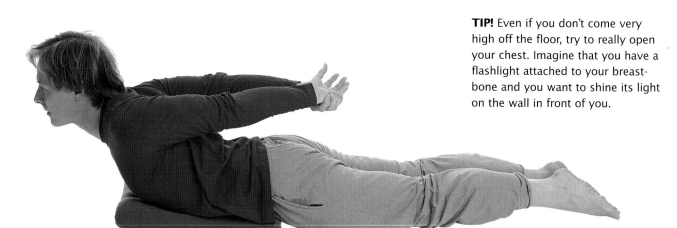

Transition: A moment's rest in Child's Pose.

NOTE: *If you've ever done yoga, you'll be familiar with one version of Child's Pose or another. Push up from the prone position and, leaving your palms flat on the floor, draw your hips back toward your heels (if you can, bring your butt to your heels). Rest your forehead on the floor and let your torso relax toward your thighs. Inhale and feel your body fill with air. Exhale and feel it sink toward the floor.*

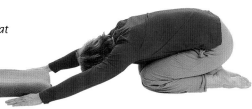

Legs: The Side Kick Series

One of my students likes to call these the "supermodel side kicks." As you go through the moves, imagine that your legs have a strong, stretchy quality and are anchored at your navel. The rhythm should be brisk but controlled. Keep the abdominals pulling in and up and reach your legs far across the room—make them supermodel long! If you are really using your abdominals, your body, from hips to head, should remain completely still as the working leg does its thing. Remember, you are working for length and strength here.

Do the entire Side Kick Series with your left leg on top first and then repeat it using the right leg. It isn't unusual for one leg to be stronger than the other. If you notice this, do the routine with the weaker leg first, then the stronger leg—and then go back to the weaker leg for another round. They'll even out if you stick with it.

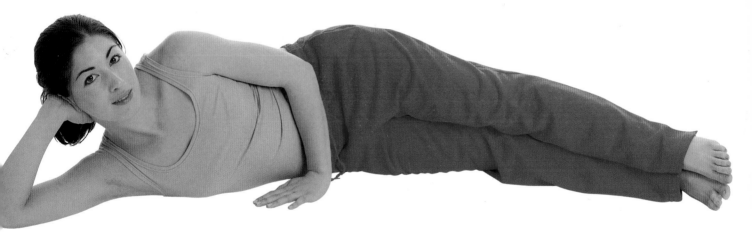

Starting position for Side Kicks: Lie on your right side, propping yourself up on your right elbow. (If this is uncomfortable, check out the position for Side Kicks in the Fix-Its section, page TK.) Place your left hand firmly on the floor in front of your belly. Your upper body, from hips to head, should be in one straight line and energized, not relaxed or slumpy. Your legs should shoot out in front of you about 20 degrees or so. And the line of your hips should be perpendicular to the floor.

SIDE KICKS FRONT/BACK

- Lift your top leg 2 or 3 inches so it's perfectly in line with the top hip socket. Kick your leg toward your nose and pulse once it is at the end of your range, then stretch your leg to the back. Exhale as you kick to

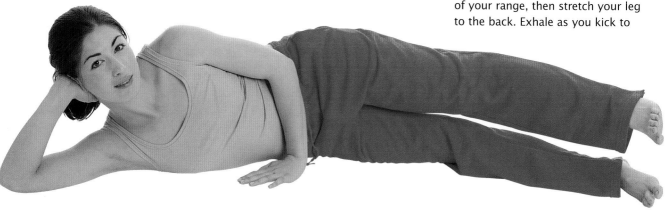

the front; inhale as you stretch to the back.

- Kick only as far as you can while keeping your hips still. Remember, a strong powerhouse will help!

- If you can concentrate on something extra, flex your foot as you

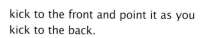

kick to the front and point it as you kick to the back.

- Do 10 Front/Backs.

- Switch sides.

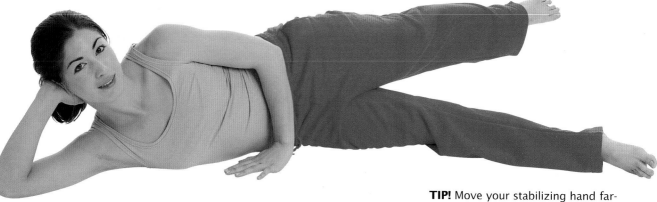

TIP! Move your stabilizing hand farther away from your body if you need extra support.

SIDE KICKS UP/DOWN

- Turn your legs out so your heels are touching. Kick your top leg toward your ear with as much freedom as you feel in your hip socket. Then, as if you're moving through peanut butter, press the leg back down. That's a quick kick up, then resistance on the way down. Inhale as the leg goes up; exhale as you press it down.

- Stretch your leg out longer and longer each time you press it down. Stretch your spine more too.

- If you want to, you can flex your foot on the way up and point it on the way down.

- Do 5 Up/Downs.

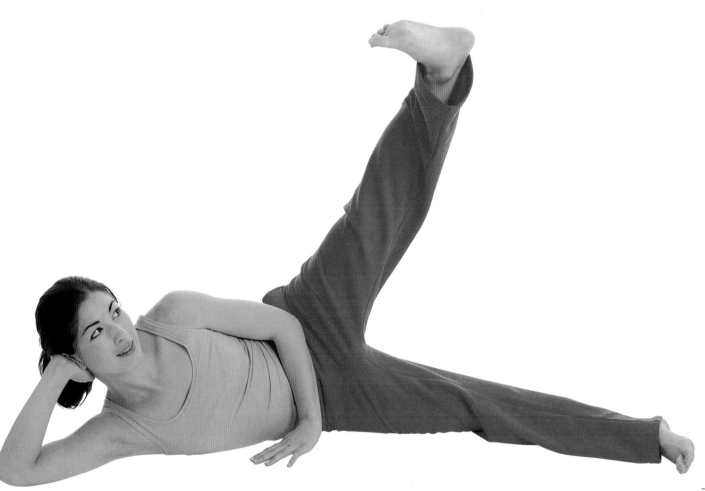

TIP! If you're wobbling around, bend your supporting leg (the one on the floor) to a 90-degree angle and point the knee out in front of your body.

LITTLE (EVIL) CIRCLES

- Keeping your leg turned out and all your parts in alignment—and I mean perfect and still—make an itty-bitty perfect circle with your top heel. Think of drawing the outline of a bubble directly above your bottom heel. Breathe naturally.

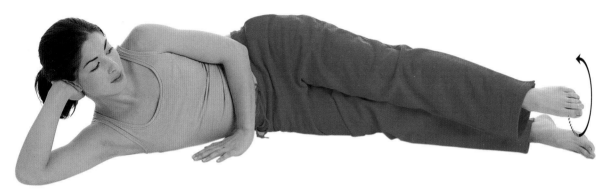

- It surprises most everyone how evil this seemingly benign exercise is. The circles can be so intense for the muscles that act around the hip and butt when you do them without moving anything else. And perfect circles are really hard to perform!

- Do 5 circles in one direction and 5 in the other.

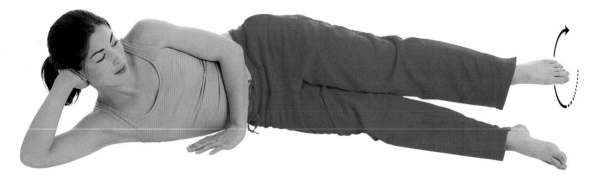

TIP! If you feel clumsy (and you're not alone—it's quite common), start with circles the size of a basketball and gradually make them smaller.

BEATS

- Shift your legs so they form a straight line with your torso. Extend your lower arm out straight and rest your head on it.

- Keeping your hips aligned and your belly pulled in and up, lift the top leg 6 inches. Hold it still and bring the bottom leg up to meet it for 5 little beats. Bring both legs down together.

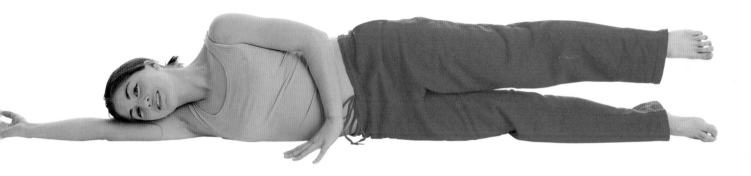

- Inhale as the top leg goes up, hold the breath for the beats, and exhale as you lower down.

- Do not tip forward or backward! Don't sacrifice placement to get the legs higher; take it lower if you need to.

- Do 5 Beats.

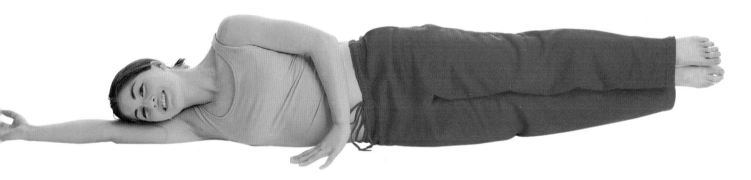

Transition: Roll over to your other side and do the Side Kick Series with your other leg. When you're finished, roll onto your back. And, by the way, nice legs!

The Final Hurdle

This series is quite challenging, but if you've done the earlier exercises with proper alignment, a strong powerhouse, and fully stretched limbs, you'll be prepared. What makes the movements so hard is the coordination, flexibility, and strength they require. To help you get through the hardest ones, I offer the following advice: Keep the focus on your abdominals and remember to commit your entire body to your movements. This, too, will get easier with practice.

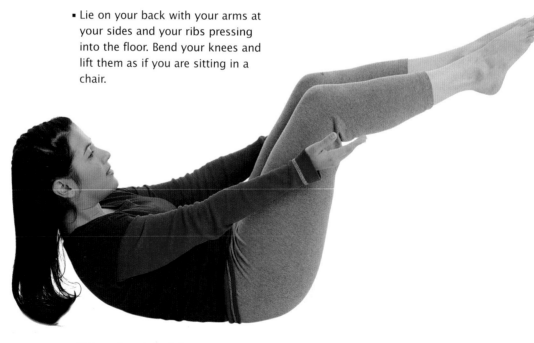

THE TEASER

- Lie on your back with your arms at your sides and your ribs pressing into the floor. Bend your knees and lift them as if you are sitting in a chair.

- Take a deep breath in to prepare, then exhale to "peel" yourself off the floor until you are balancing at the point just behind your tailbone.

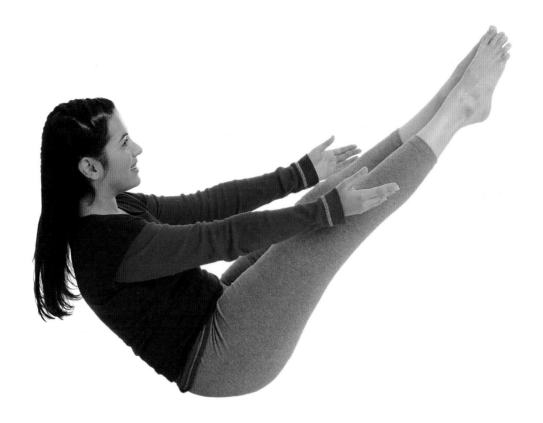

- Press your arms and legs through space so they're fully outstretched at the time when you hit that balance.

- Pause and inhale. Exhale as you roll back down to the floor with control.

- Move as slowly and fluidly as you can. Think of your spine getting longer each time you roll down.

- Do 5 Teasers.

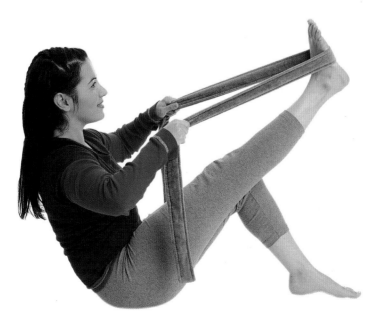

TIP! This one is hard. A great modification is to try it with one foot on the floor and a strap around the raised leg.

Transition: Bring your feet to the floor and extend your body completely. Roll over onto your belly so you're like a superhero flying through the air.

SWIMMING

- I must warn you that many people hate this exercise! It's very challenging—and, of course, so good for you. Without scrunching the back of your neck, raise your head. Lift your right arm and your left leg off the floor simultaneously. Remember: belly pulled in and up.

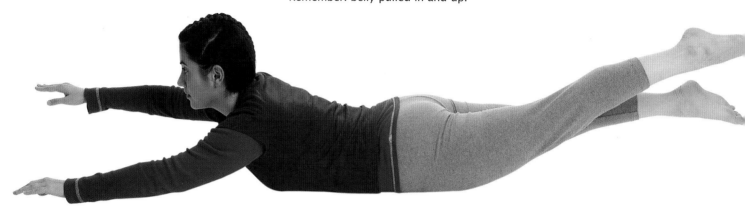

- Now "swim" briskly above the surface of the floor, changing back and forth from right arm, left leg up to left arm, right leg up. Once you've begun, your feet and hands never touch the ground.

- Inhale and swim for 8 counts; exhale and swim for 8 counts. (Each side change is a count.)

- Do this for 3 breaths.

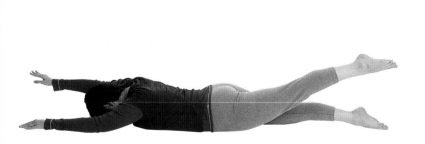

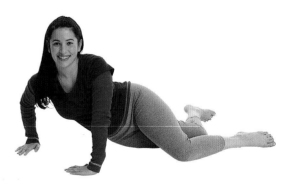

TIP! This can be really awkward if your back is weak or the muscles on one side of your body are underdeveloped. To make it more manageable, leave your head down and do the arm and leg work slowly, allowing the resting limbs to remain on the floor.

Transition: Roll onto your right side and push yourself to sitting on your right hip. Pull your heels in to the left side of your hips, knees pointing straight ahead.

THE MERMAID

- This exercise consists of two delicious side stretches. For the first one, hold your left ankle with your left hand. Take your right arm up to the ceiling. Exhale and bend toward your feet. Inhale to come back to sitting tall.

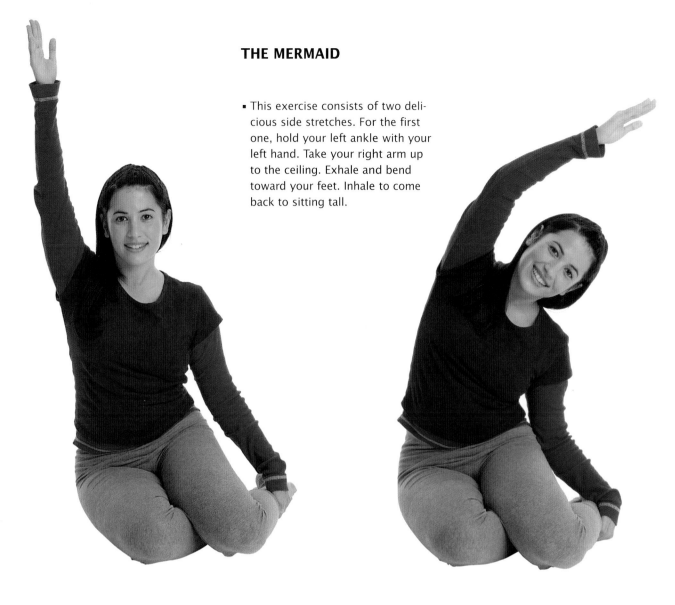

- For the second stretch, place your right elbow on the floor, fingertips pointing away from your feet.

Exhale and stretch away from your feet, reaching your left arm over your head. In this position, your supporting arm should be really active so you don't slouch into your shoulder. Inhale to come back to sitting tall.

- Throughout the entire exercise—even between the two stretches—think "long, long, LONG!"

- Do 3 Mermaids sitting on your right hip.

- To change sides, stretch the legs forward, then bring your heels to the right side of your hips.

- Do 3 Mermaids sitting on your left hip.

TIP! If this is hard on your knees, place a pillow or folded blanket under the hip you're sitting on.

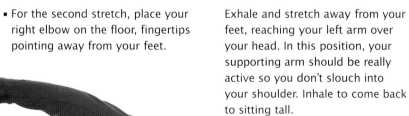

Transition: Lie facedown with your hands at your sides.

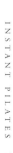

PREP FOR ROCKING

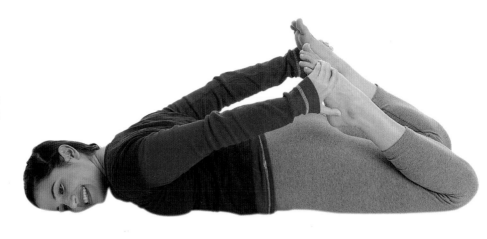

- Bend your knees and reach back to grab your ankles. If it's enough just to hold this position, stop there and breathe.

- To continue, push your ankles into your hands. This will help you lift your head and chest off the floor. Allow your shoulders and chest to open up as you keep pushing with your feet.

- Hold this position for 3 breaths.

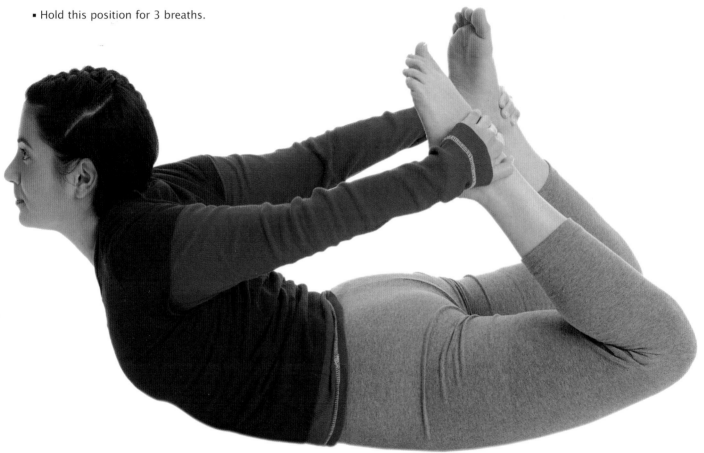

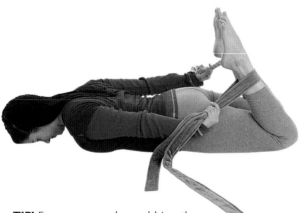

TIP! For some people, grabbing the ankles is extremely hard. If this is the case, loop a strap around each ankle and hold the ends.

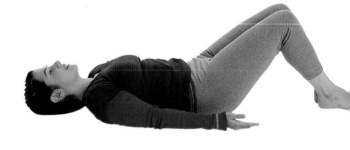

Transition: Press back into Child's Pose (see page TK), then roll over onto your back with your knees bent.

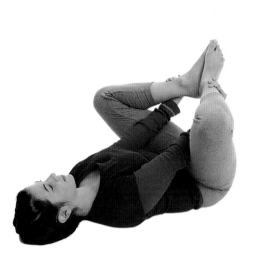
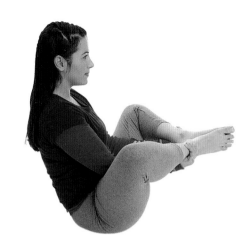
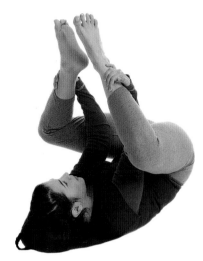

THE SEAL

- Draw your feet in toward your chest, knees turned out. Take a full breath.

- Lift your head and shoulders off the floor and rock up to a sitting balance. Clap your feet together 3 times the way a seal claps, then rock back to your shoulders. Clap 3 times while balancing there.

- Rock back and forth in a smooth, controlled way.

- The claps are a release for your hips and force you to maintain enough control to fit them in. You must control the roll; it can't control you.

- Inhale as you rock back to the shoulders; exhale as you come up.

- Do 5 Seals.

TIP! If this is too difficult, hold your legs under your thighs—but keep the claps!

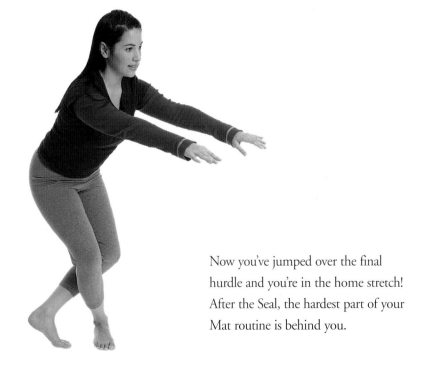

Transition: You may have to work up to this one. Release your feet and roll forward once more. This time, bring your feet to the floor, crossing one foot in front of the other to rise to standing—this is one of the few Pilates moves where you are encouraged to use momentum this way! As your feet hit the floor, think of sending your head forward and up. It can feel strange at first, but you'll get it with practice.

Now you've jumped over the final hurdle and you're in the home stretch! After the Seal, the hardest part of your Mat routine is behind you.

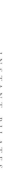

The Arm Series

The Arm Series is a great way to take everything you've learned lying down and put it to the test in the standing position. As your arms move, your core stabilizing muscles (abdominals and erector spinae) engage to keep your torso from swaying. This is what makes the Arm Series an essential component of your Mat routine. Throughout all these exercises, pretend that you're pressing against an imaginary force to create your own resistance. If you want to make it more challenging, use light weights (2 or 3 pounds) or even canned vegetables.

Starting position for the Arm Series: Stand with your legs together, feet slightly turned out so they make a small V. Keep the legs feeling long and strong and, as always, pull your belly in and up. Squeeze the muscles in your butt to help stabilize the pelvis. Remember also to relax the neck and shoulders. Think of your shoulder blades sliding down your back like warm butter—not popping up toward your ears! Check your alignment: Ears, shoulders, hips, knees, and ankles should all be stacked one on top of the other from the side view.

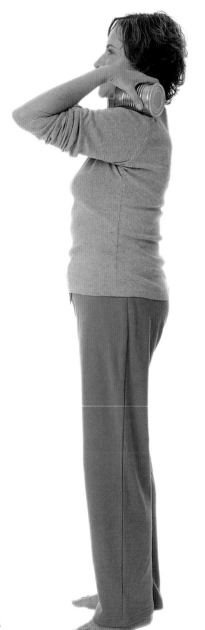
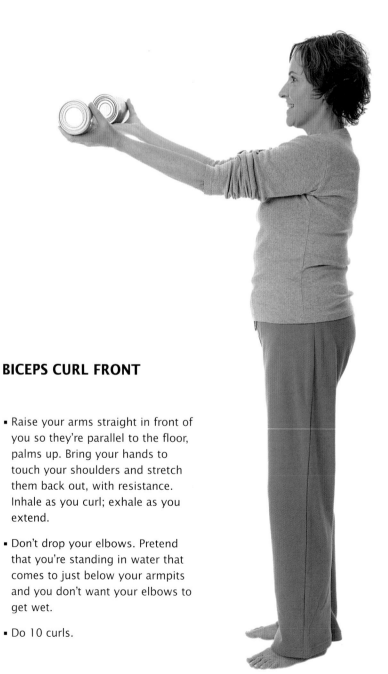

BICEPS CURL FRONT

- Raise your arms straight in front of you so they're parallel to the floor, palms up. Bring your hands to touch your shoulders and stretch them back out, with resistance. Inhale as you curl; exhale as you extend.

- Don't drop your elbows. Pretend that you're standing in water that comes to just below your armpits and you don't want your elbows to get wet.

- Do 10 curls.

BICEPS CURL SIDE

- Take your arms out to the sides. If you look straight ahead they should still be in your peripheral vision.

- Curl and uncurl as for Biceps Curl Front. Exhale bringing the arms in; inhale pressing them out with resistance.

- Remember—no wet elbows, neck and shoulders relaxed. Are you still pulling your belly button to your spine?

- Do 10 curls.

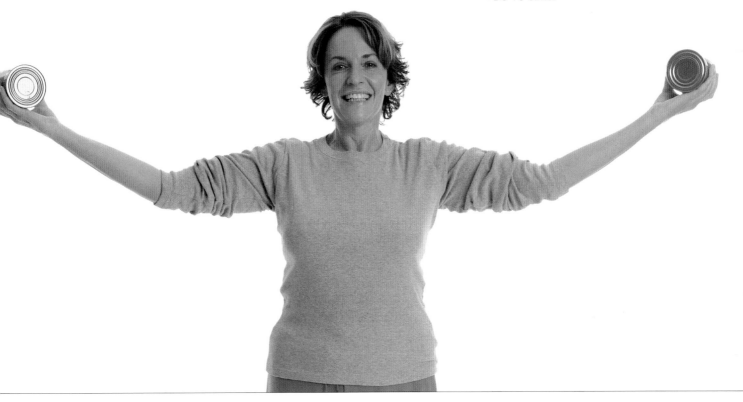

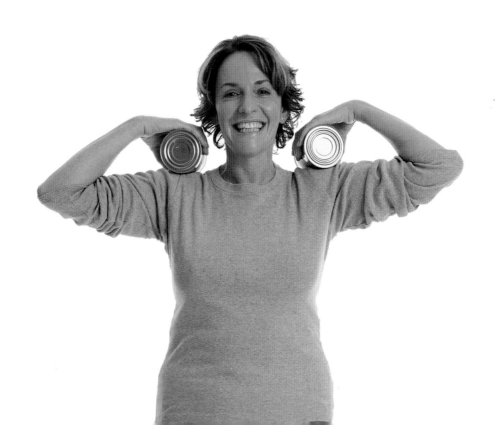

CHICKEN WINGS

- Point your elbows as far behind you as you can and, if you are not holding weights, make fists.

- Moving only from the elbows down, press your lower arms behind you to extend your arms. Exhale as you press and extend; inhale as you bend.

- Do 10 repetitions.

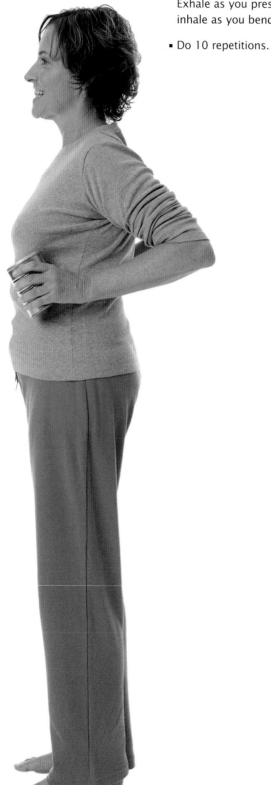

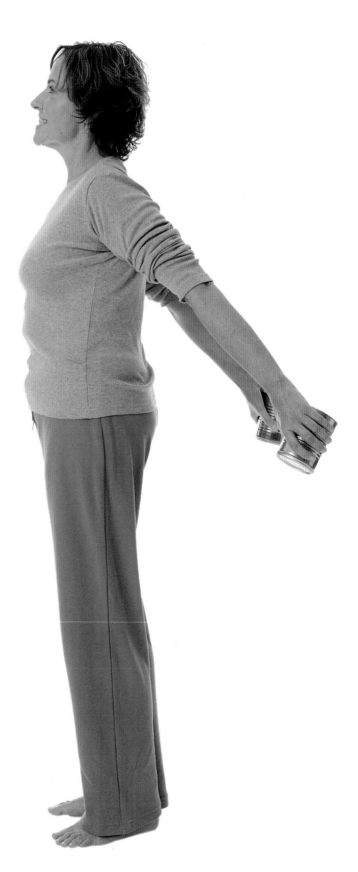

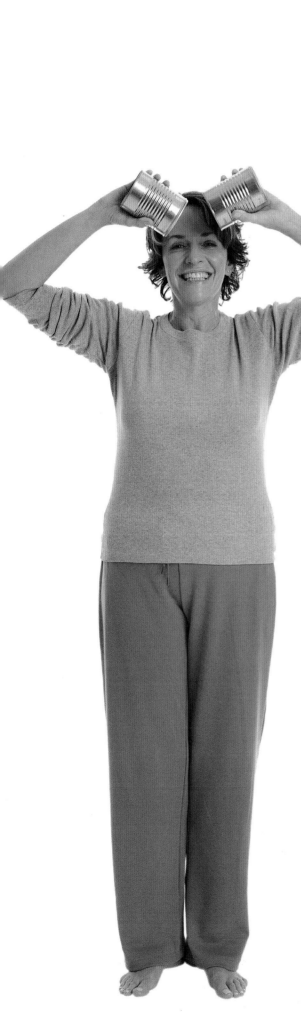

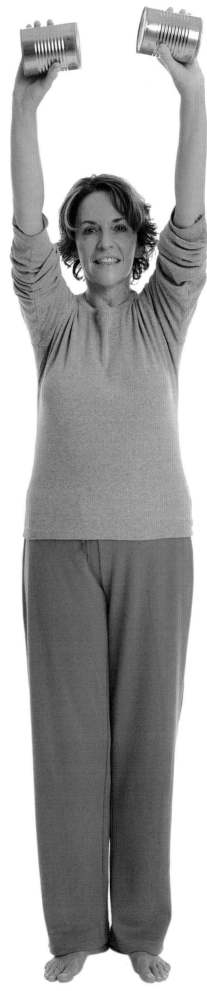

SALUTES

- Bring your hands to your forehead, with your elbows to the sides in a double salute.

- Stretch your arms up and slightly forward, then bend your elbows to return to the starting position, taking care to aim them toward the side walls again. Exhale as you extend; inhale as you return.

- Try not to bonk yourself in the head with your weights (happens all the time)!

- Do 10 Salutes.

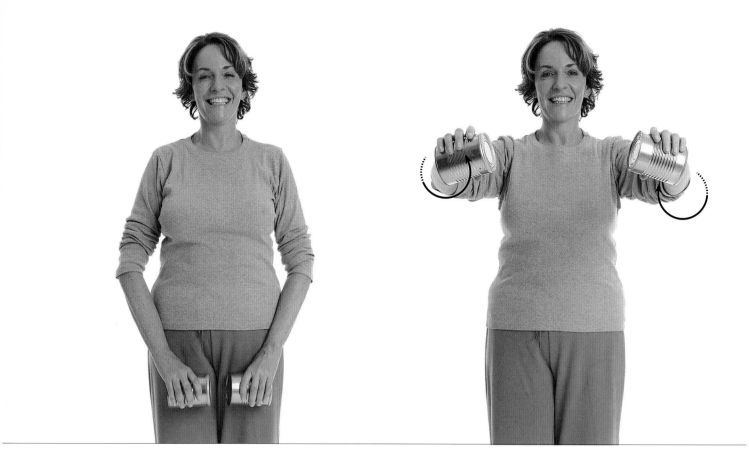

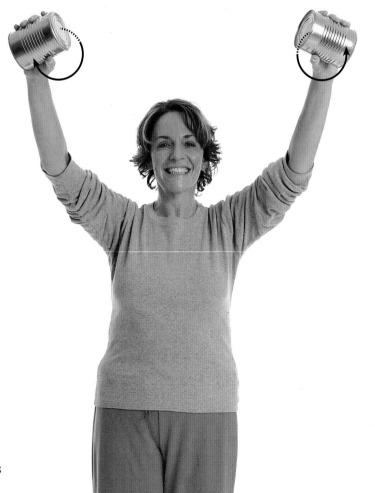

CIRCLES

- Start with your arms at your sides, elbows slightly bent. Make 10 quick little circles as you raise your arms in front of you, reaching all the way up to the sky. Reverse the circles on the way back down. Inhale as you go up; exhale on the way down.

- Keep your stabilizing muscles (abs, butt, inner thighs) active so your body doesn't wiggle as your arms circle.

- Do 5 sets.

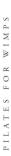

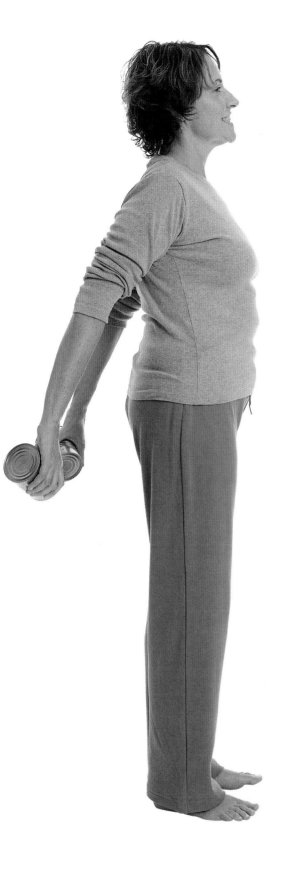
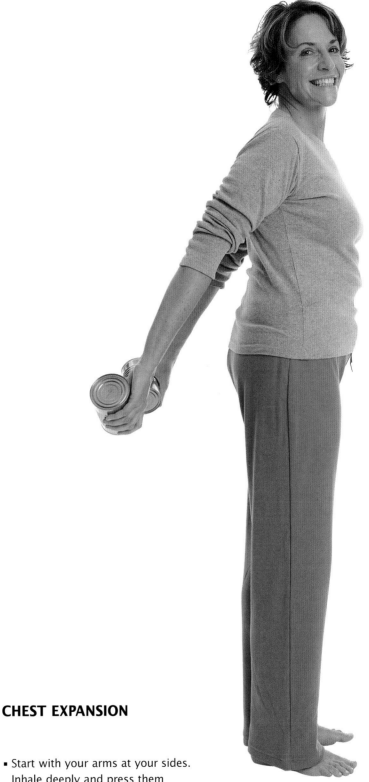

CHEST EXPANSION

- Start with your arms at your sides. Inhale deeply and press them behind you, drawing the shoulder blades together. Think of cracking a walnut between your shoulder blades.

- Hold the breath and turn your head first to the right, then to the left. Center your head, then exhale as you release your arms.

- Do 6 Chest Expansions, alternating the side you look to first.

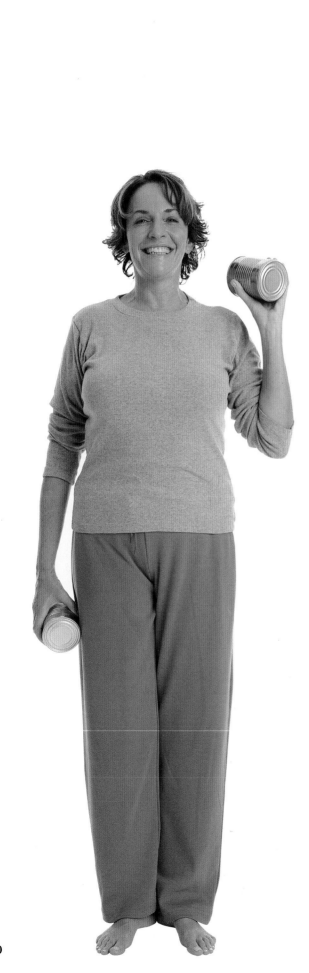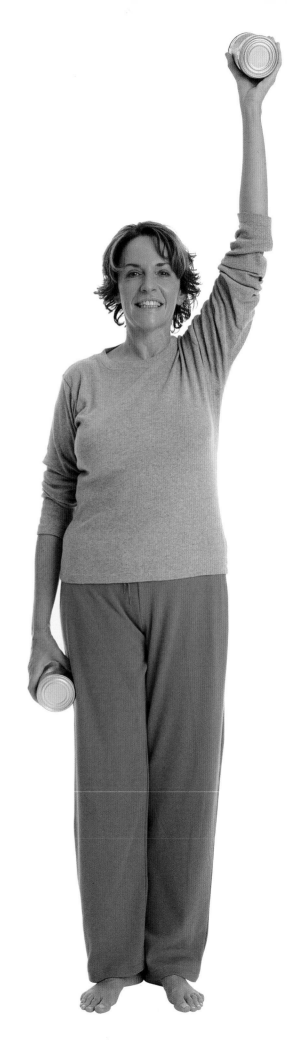

SIDE STRETCH

- Bring your left weight (or your hand, if you're not using weights) in toward your left shoulder, then inhale and stretch your arm all the way up to the ceiling. Exhale and side bend to the right.

- Let your right arm hang by your side, and think of getting super-long from your left foot to your left fingertips.

- Inhale to come back up to standing. Exhale and bring the left arm back down the way it came up—bending through the elbow.

- Change sides and do the same thing, bending to the left.

- Do 6 stretches (3 on each side).

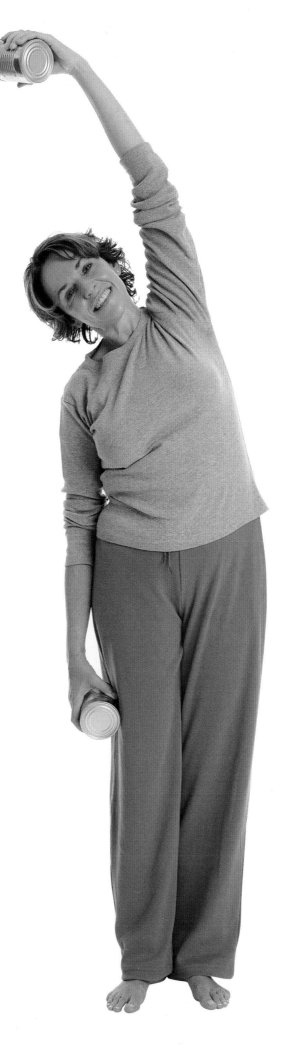

The Wall to Finish

This series is pure genius in its simplicity and effectiveness. It's a wonderful thing to do anytime. I recommend it highly and frequently to anyone who sits at a desk, carries kids around, or has muscle imbalance or scoliosis. As a matter of fact, when I'm done writing this section, I am going to go do the Wall. But as an ending to your Mat work, it also serves as a time to gently move through space with breath, length, and symmetry. I was originally going to say it's like the period at the end of a sentence—but since Pilates stays with you after you've finished the routine, it's really more like ellipsis points . . .

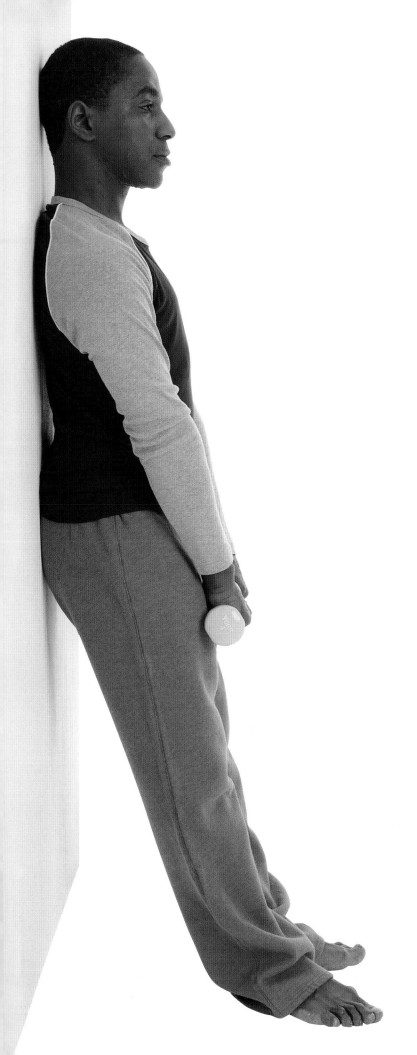

Starting position for the Wall:
Stand with your back against a wall, feet slightly turned out to form a V and about a foot away from the wall. Your spine is in a neutral position, with the back of your pelvis, ribs, shoulder blades, and head touching the wall. Your arms are hanging in front, palms toward you, hands or weights touching. (You can do the series with or without light weights.)

TIP! If you have very rounded shoulders and have trouble getting your head to touch the wall, place a pillow or a book behind your head so it is comfortably supported.

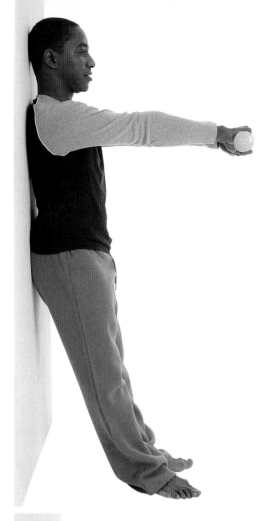

WIDE ARM CIRCLES

- Slowly reach the arms forward and up toward the sky, then out toward the sides of the room and back to the starting position.

- Look straight ahead and keep your hands just inside your peripheral vision. Inhale as the arms go up; exhale as they come down.

- Do 3 circles in one direction, then reverse for 3.

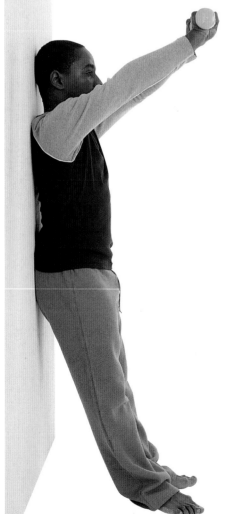

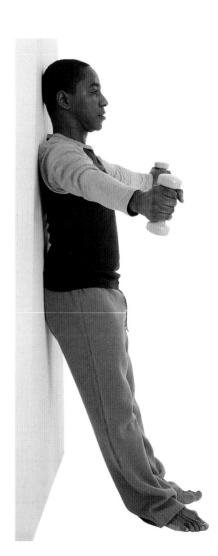

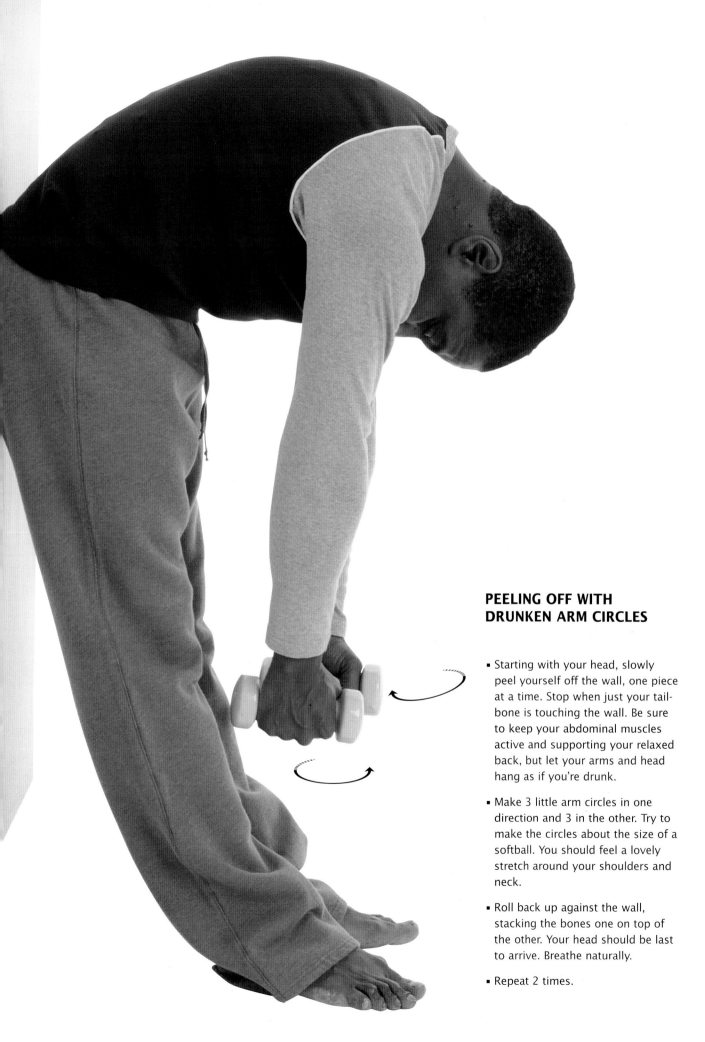

PEELING OFF WITH DRUNKEN ARM CIRCLES

- Starting with your head, slowly peel yourself off the wall, one piece at a time. Stop when just your tail-bone is touching the wall. Be sure to keep your abdominal muscles active and supporting your relaxed back, but let your arms and head hang as if you're drunk.

- Make 3 little arm circles in one direction and 3 in the other. Try to make the circles about the size of a softball. You should feel a lovely stretch around your shoulders and neck.

- Roll back up against the wall, stacking the bones one on top of the other. Your head should be last to arrive. Breathe naturally.

- Repeat 2 times.

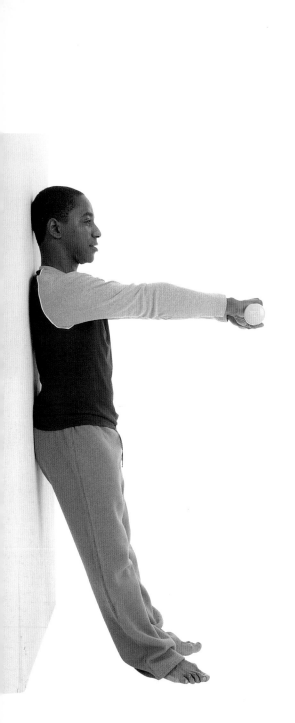

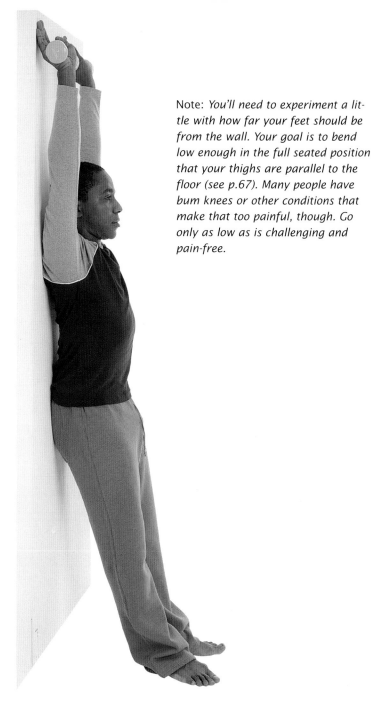

Note: *You'll need to experiment a little with how far your feet should be from the wall. Your goal is to bend low enough in the full seated position that your thighs are parallel to the floor (see p.67). Many people have bum knees or other conditions that make that too painful, though. Go only as low as is challenging and pain-free.*

WALL TOUCHES

- This might turn out to be your favorite Pilates exercise. It feels great, it's super-simple, and you can do it anytime. Inhale and reach your arms forward and up to touch the wall behind you. Exhale and bring the arms back down to your sides.

- You should feel a nice stretch in your upper body wherever you happen to hold tension. If your ribs start to come off the wall, stop there and try to press them back while pressing your arms into the wall, too.

- Do 5 Wall Touches.

Transition: If you've been supporting your head with an accessory, set it aside. Open your legs so they are hip-width apart. Point your toes straight ahead and move your feet far enough from the wall that when you "sit," your lower legs are perpendicular to the floor.

SITTING

- Keeping your back against the wall, slide downward until your butt is just above the height of your knees (or until you have gone as far as you can). Remember, your lower legs should be perpendicular to the floor. As you slide, raise your arms just as you did in Wall Touches.

- Hold for 5 counts and slide back up.

- Inhale as you go down; hold the breath as you sit; exhale as you return to the starting position.

- Do 3 Sittings.

Congratulations! You have completed a full Pilates Mat routine. It gets smoother and easier each time you do it. When you're ready, flip to the Bonus Points! section. You'll see new, more difficult exercises, as well as more challenging versions of some exercises you've already done. But make no mistake, the routine you've just learned will keep your body long, strong, flexible, and balanced.

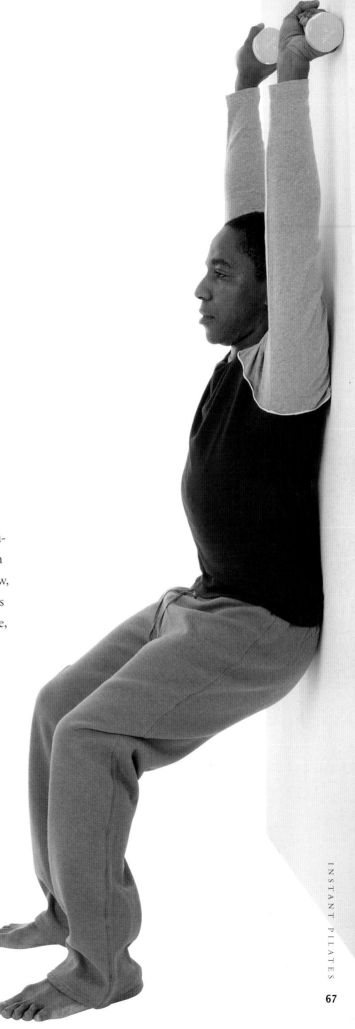

The following pages bring you different Pilates menus for everyday body/mind hungers. Whether you need to re-energize after a tiresome day, boost yourself out of a gloomy mood, squeeze a quickie Mat routine into your crazy morning, or take a body break from the desk, you'll find a short and sweet section to soothe you. Some of the exercises are ones you've already seen—classic Mat exercises pulled out for a specific benefit. Some are Pilates exercises that aren't part of the Mat routine but are still tremendously beneficial for a particular bug. A very few are modifications of classic exercises that I've come up with for fun and functionality.

2
Fix-Its

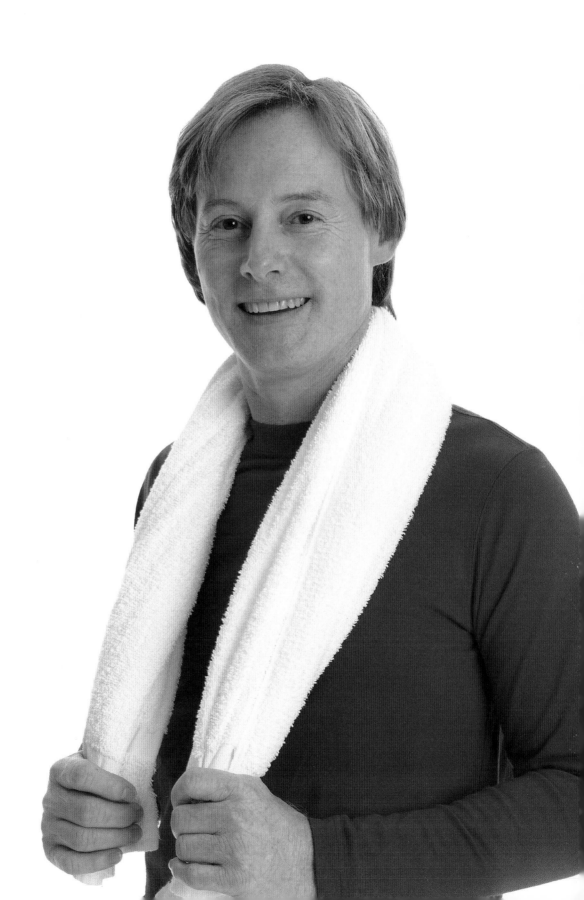

The Computer Blues

There aren't too many things that can be worse for your body than sitting at a desk and staring at a computer terminal. I love my computer, but staring . . . waiting . . . clicking . . . typing . . . reading . . . scrolling . . . staring, even for just 30 minutes, whether for work or for play, is completely unnatural. It brings on a ton of muscle strain to sit still and hunched, gazing intently at a glowing screen. What can you do about it? Take a break! You don't have to do all these exercises to reap the benefits. When you notice you've been still for even 15 minutes, do just one. If you've been there for an hour, do them all! If your boss catches you, just remind her of the money you're saving the company by staying healthy!

There's also a lot you can do to lessen strain when you're trapped at your desk. As ever, proper alignment is the key—the same alignment you practice in sitting exercises. Here are some guidelines for a healthful sitting posture:

1. Balance your head over your shoulders.
2. Balance your shoulders over your hips.
3. Allow your lower back to have a slight natural curve inward.
4. Aim your sit bones directly toward the floor.
5. Keep your knees pointing straight ahead and hip-width apart.

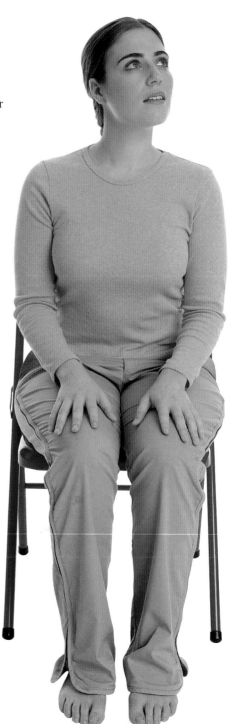

NOSE CIRCLES

- Slowly draw 3 clockwise circles, then 3 counterclockwise circles, with your nose.

- Concentrate on hitting every point of a perfect circle, breathe naturally, and keep the rest of your body still.

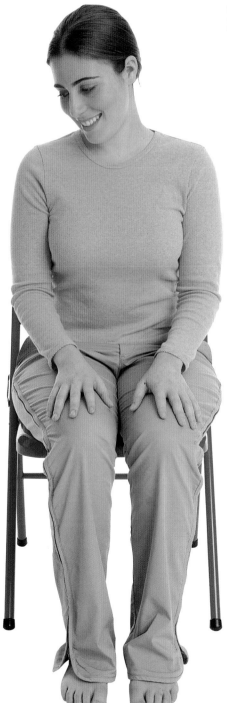
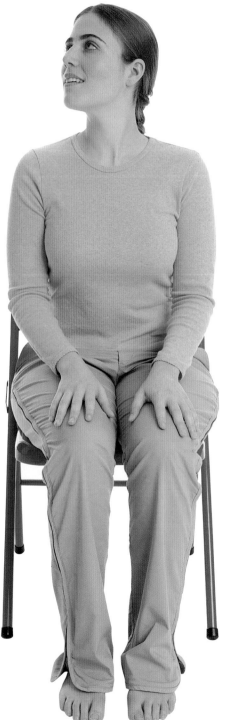

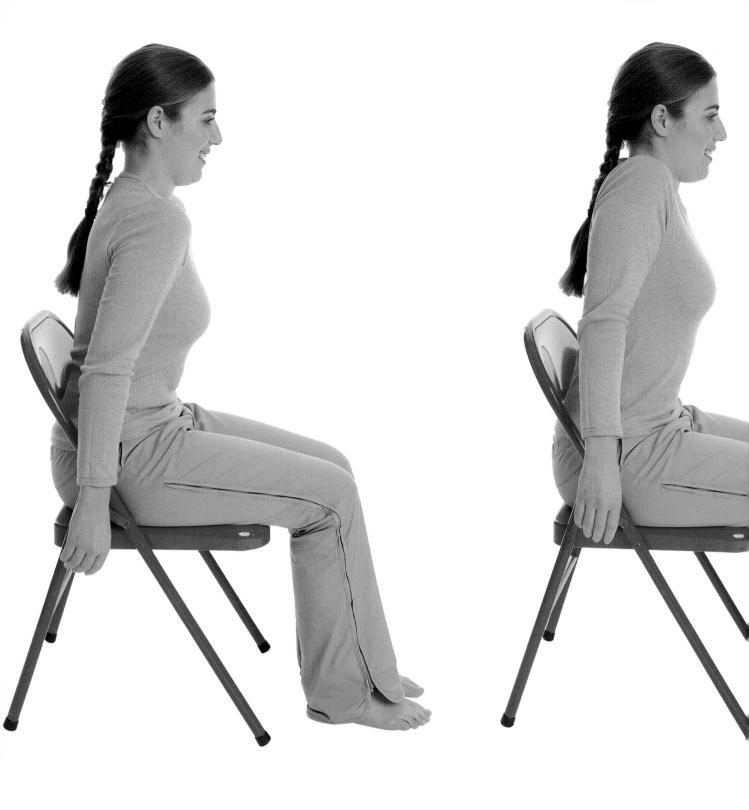

SHOULDER ROLLS

- Roll your shoulders forward, up, back, and down. Do 3 rolls, then reverse for 3.

- Again, visualize a perfect circle, breathe naturally, and keep your body still.

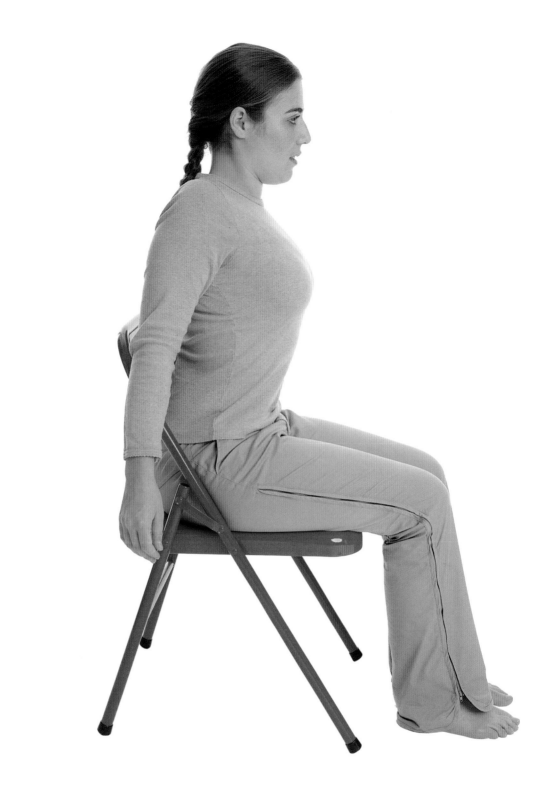

SHAVING THE BACK OF THE HEAD

- Lean forward very slightly but keep your torso as straight as possible from head to tailbone. Your abdominals are supporting your back. Bring your hands to the base of your skull, elbows pointing out.

- Inhale and stretch your arms out along an imaginary diagonal line, grazing the back of your head, until they are fully extended. Exhale and return your arms to the starting position, keeping your elbows angled outward.

- Do 10 Shavings.

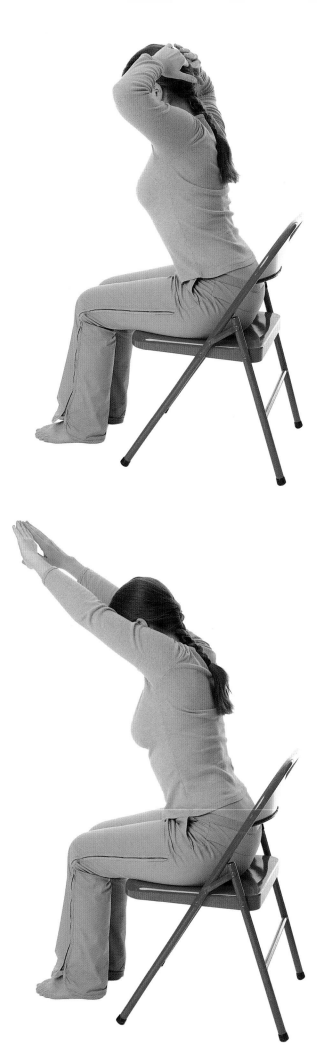

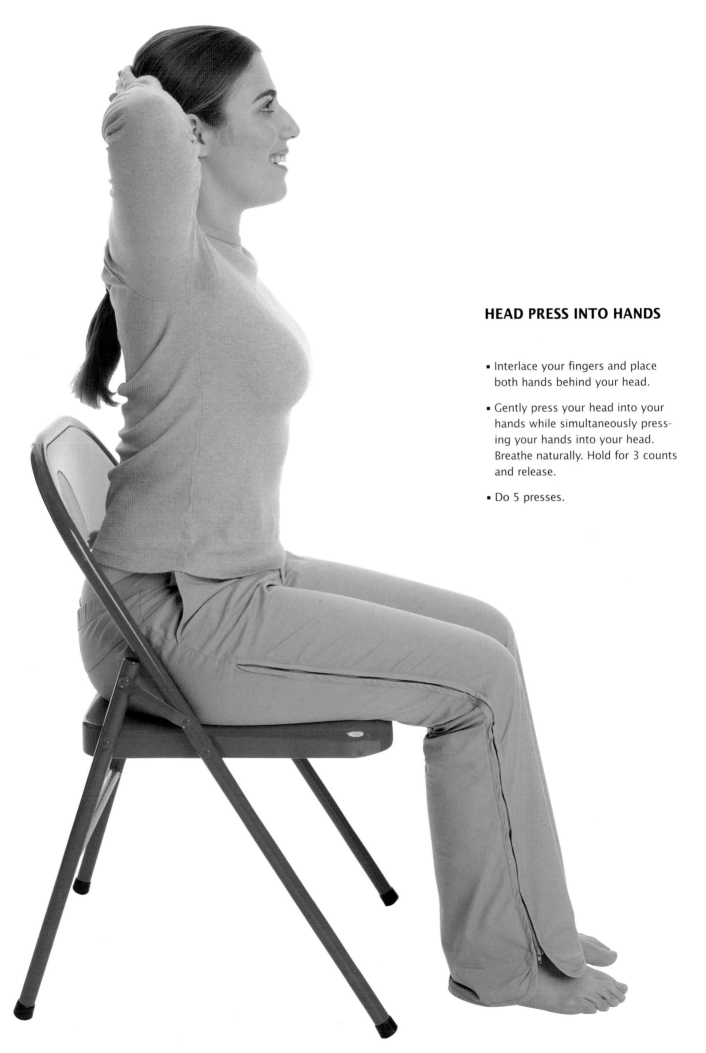

HEAD PRESS INTO HANDS

- Interlace your fingers and place both hands behind your head.

- Gently press your head into your hands while simultaneously pressing your hands into your head. Breathe naturally. Hold for 3 counts and release.

- Do 5 presses.

SUCK A LEMON/BITE AN APPLE

- This one is particularly great if you've been focusing hard with your eyes because it loosens up the facial muscles. Make a face like you've just tasted an incredibly sour lemon—squeeze every muscle in your face toward your nose.

- Next, open your mouth like you're taking an immense bite out of the hugest apple you've ever had in your life—pull all those facial muscles away from your nose.

- Breathe naturally. Just one of these is fine, but if you'd like to do more, feel free!

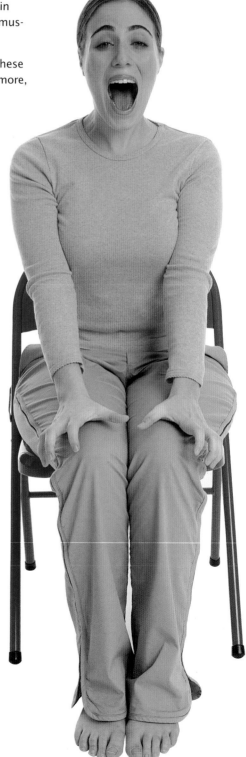

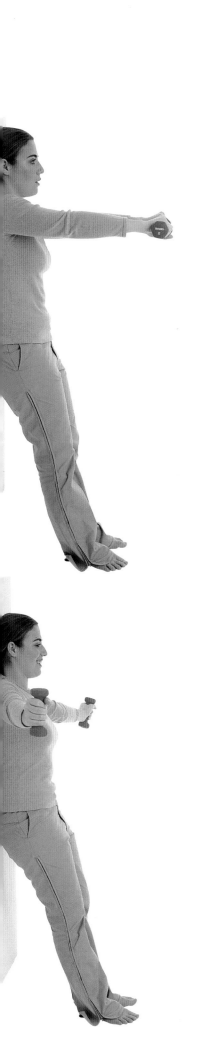

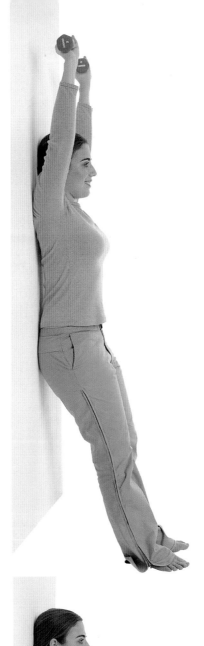

WIDE ARM CIRCLES

- Stand with your back against the wall, feet slightly turned out to form a V and about a foot away from the wall. Your arms are hanging in front, palms toward you, hands (or light weights) touching.

- Slowly reach the arms forward and up toward the sky, then out toward the sides of the room and back to the starting position.

- Look straight ahead and keep your hands just inside your peripheral vision. Inhale as the arms go up; exhale as they come down.

- Do 3 circles in one direction, then reverse for 3.

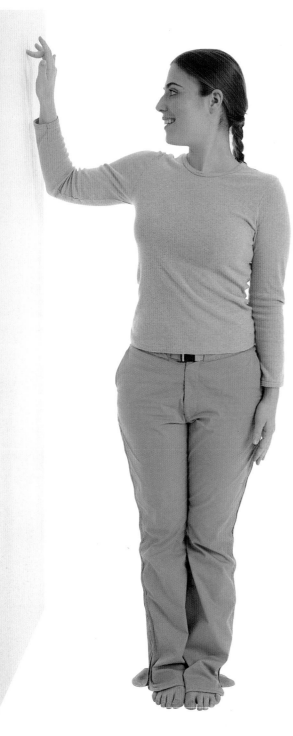
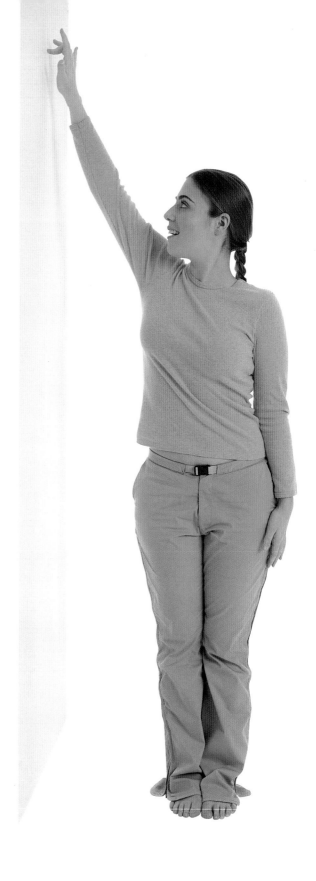

ARM CRAWL ON THE WALL

- Stand with one shoulder facing the wall, your hand on the wall in line with the shoulder and your elbow hanging straight down to the floor.

- Slowly walk your fingers up the wall until your arm is extended. Then walk your fingers back down. Be sure to keep your elbow aiming toward the floor the entire time.

- Inhale as you stretch up; exhale as you come down.

- Do this once looking at your hand, then once looking straight ahead.

- Turn and repeat on the opposite side.

Neck, Shoulder, and Lower Back Lock-Up

It appears that the shoulder girdle and the pelvic girdle are partners in crime. They both help to support and carry major loads, and if you have tension around one, the other doesn't want to feel left out. I've had clients with intense neck and jaw tension, and when I stretch out the muscles surrounding the pelvis, the tension in their upper body is released. If you have any ruckus going on from your hips to your head, this section will turn it into sweet harmony.

CHILD'S POSE ON YOUR CHAIR

- Place a pillow on your lap and flop over like a rag doll, allowing your arms to dangle straight down.

- Take deep 3 breaths.

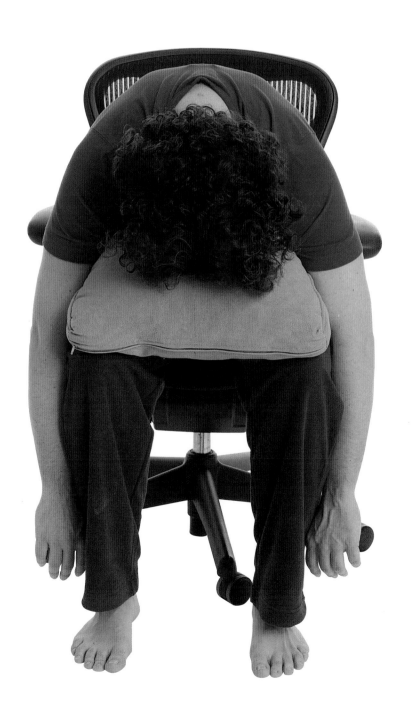

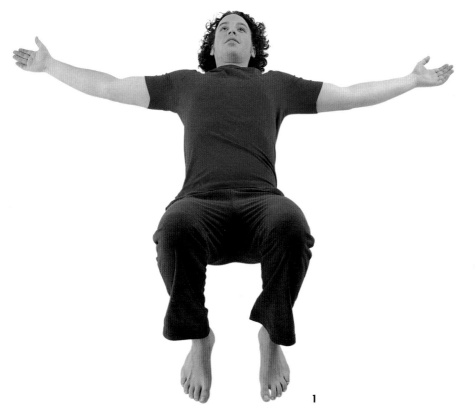

CHALK CIRCLES

- Lie on your back, arms out to the sides of the room, knees bent and hip-width apart. Let your legs fall to the right and turn your head to the left.

1

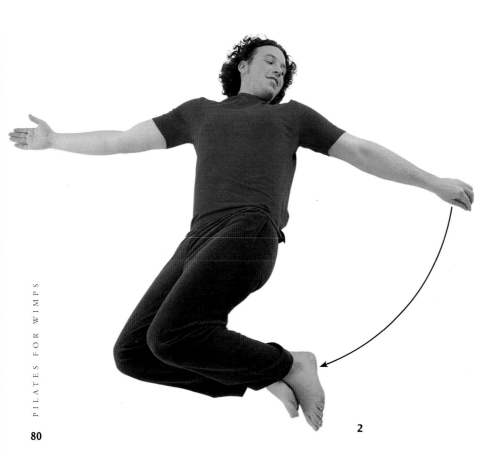

- Holding an imaginary piece of chalk in your left hand, slowly draw a circle around your body, as far as your arm can reach. Keep your hand touching the floor for as much of the circle as possible. Keep your neck muscles relaxed by allowing your head to rest on the floor the entire time. Breathe deeply.

2

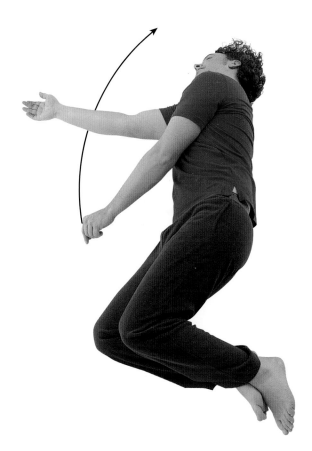

3

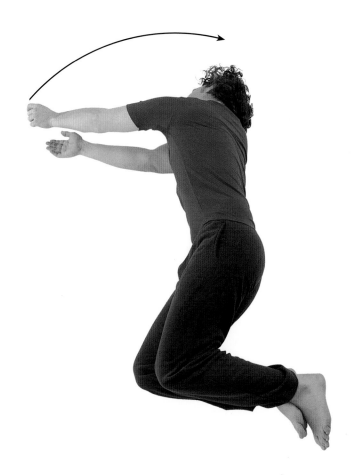

- Make 3 circles in one direction, then 3 in the other.

- Switch sides.

4

WIDE ARM CIRCLES ON THE FLOOR

- This is wonderful with or without weight. Lie with your knees bent, feet about hip-width apart. Place a pillow or blanket under you, running from your shoulders to your tailbone. Keep your abdominals

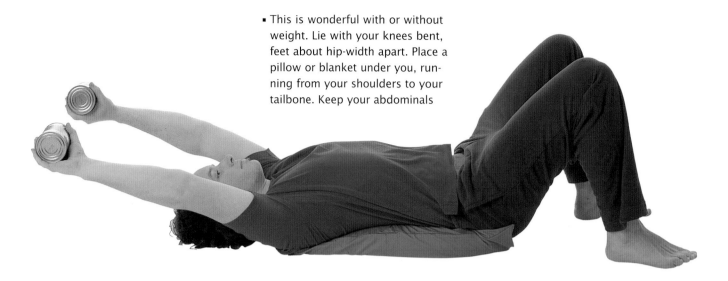

active so that your ribs don't stick out whenever you bring your arms up.

- Slowly circle the weights (or your hands) within your peripheral vision. Inhale as your arms pass over your body; exhale as they sweep out to the sides.

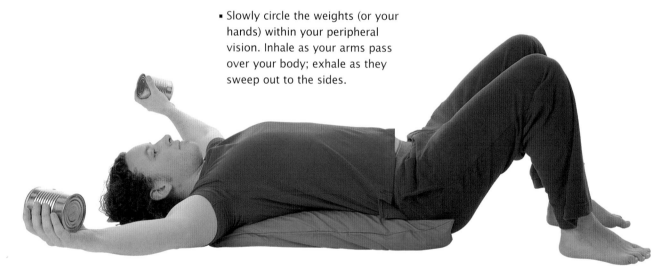

- Circle 3 times in one direction and 3 in the other.

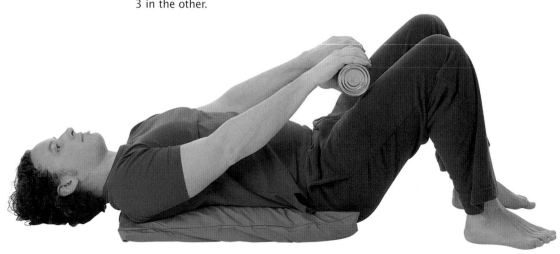

SINKING SPHINX

- Lie on your tummy and prop your-self up with your arms, placing your elbows directly under your shoulders so that your upper arms are perpendicular to the floor.

- Inhale, maintaining the position while actively pressing into the floor with your forearms. Visualize your shoulder blades moving away from each other as you press.

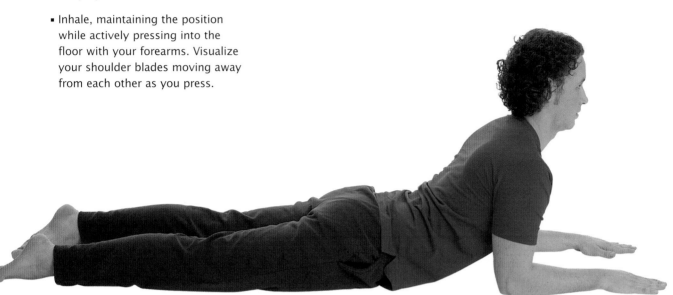

- Exhale and let your body sink, thinking of your shoulder blades moving toward each other.

- As you press and sink, the muscles acting on your shoulder blades lengthen and contract. It's like a massage for the muscles around your neck and shoulders.

- Do 8 Sinking Sphinxes.

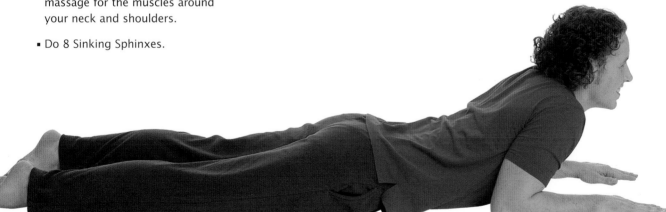

BALLET STRETCHES FRONT

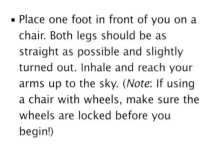

- Place one foot in front of you on a chair. Both legs should be as straight as possible and slightly turned out. Inhale and reach your arms up to the sky. (*Note*: If using a chair with wheels, make sure the wheels are locked before you begin!)

- Keeping both legs extended and your spine long, exhale and reach out over your leg. Reach toward the back of the chair and grab it, if possible, but don't sacrifice your alignment. Inhale as you return to standing.

- Do this 2 times with the legs slightly turned out and 2 times with the legs perfectly parallel.

- Go directly to the next exercise (you'll return to this stretch when you switch legs).

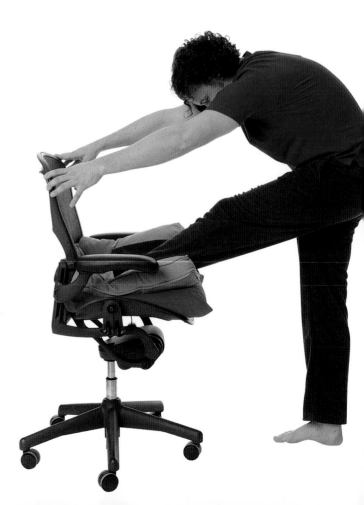

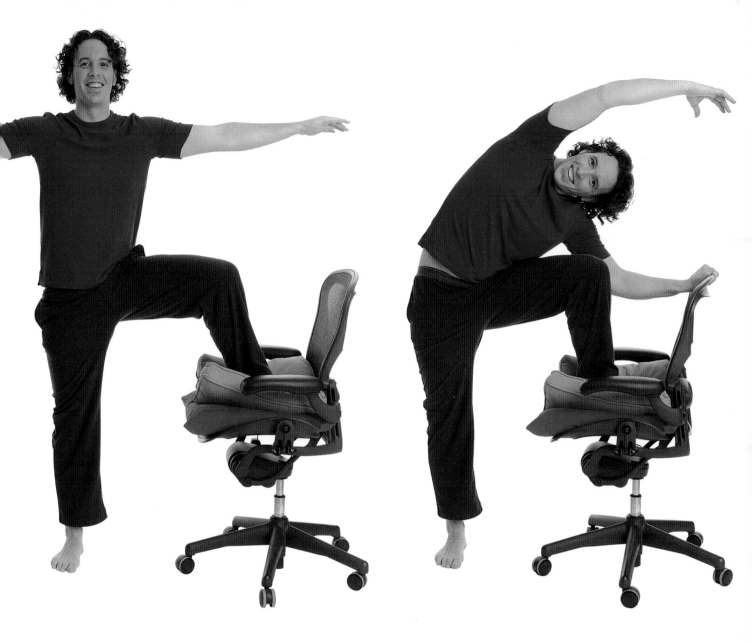

BALLET STRETCHES SIDE (FOR THE HIP)

- Turn your body so the leg on the chair is to the side. Keep your foot just within your peripheral vision as you look straight ahead. Bend your knee and place your foot flat on the chair seat. The knee and foot of your standing leg should face straight ahead of you.

- Inhale, lifting your arms to the sides. Exhale and tip sideways toward the foot on the chair, stretching your outer arm overhead toward the back of the chair while holding the back of the chair with your other hand. Inhale as you return to standing.

- Do 3 stretches.

- Switch sides and start with Ballet Stretches Front.

Mood Revitalizers

Let's face it—no matter how bubbly your natural disposition, you sometimes feel sad, bored, short-tempered, or just plain blasé. Often, though, you can make a quick mood change in just 10 minutes of focusing the mind on the body. These exercises were chosen for their general "feel-good" qualities as well as their ability to stimulate the flow of blood and oxygen get your endorphins kicking. I wouldn't be surprised if you end up feeling so good that you want to do more!

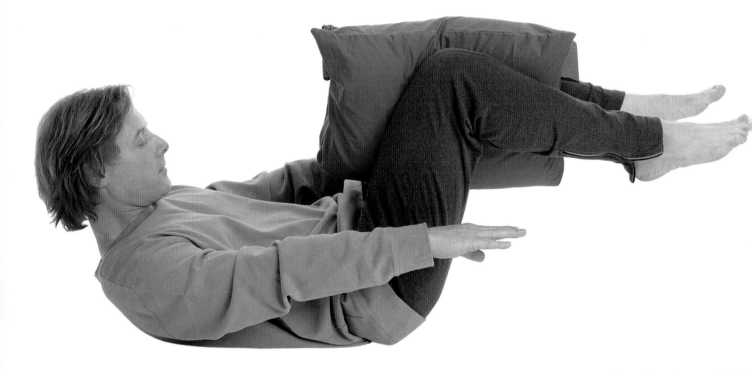

THE I-JUST-NEED-TO-GET-MYSELF-GOING HUNDRED

- Lying on your back, place a pillow between your knees and bend them in to your chest, squeezing to hold the pillow in place.

- Pull your stomach in and lift your head, shoulders, and arms off the floor. Pump your arms at your sides at a brisk tempo.

- Inhale deeply for 5 pumps; exhale completely for 5 pumps. Do this for 10 full breaths.

- I threw in the pillow for two reasons: First, you get extra credit for doing the inner thigh work to keep it there. And second, it's a fun distraction from whatever's bumming you out. You can, of course, do without it (as on page TK).

Note: *Shallow breathing usually accompanies a down mood, so all that new air is like changing the altitude. If you feel a little light-headed afterward, just rest your head on the floor and take a moment to return to your natural breath.*

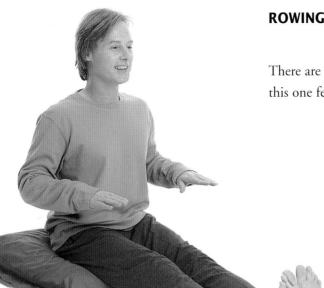

ROWING #4

There are other Pilates rowings, but this one feels the most liberating.

1

- Sit with your legs extended and together, feet flexed. Begin with a super-long spine, elbows pulled close to your sides, and forearms parallel to the floor.

2

- Inhale and bow forward over your legs.
- Exhale and extend your arms along the sides of your legs.

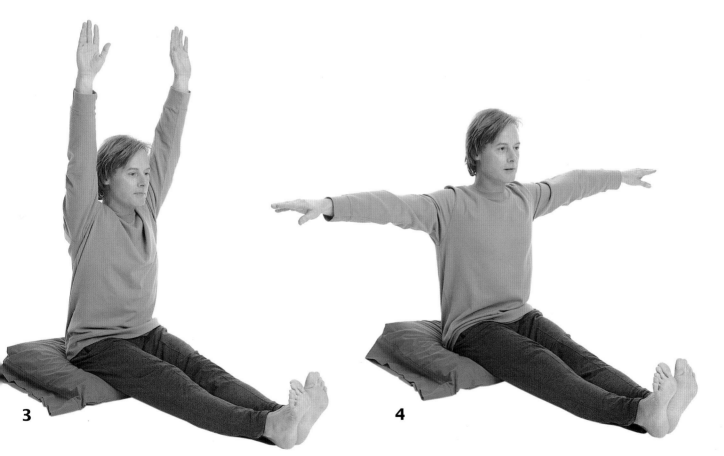

3

- Inhale while stretching back up to sitting. Bring your arms straight overhead, press your tailbone into the floor, and stack your vertebrae one on top of the other.

4

- Exhale as you open your arms out to the sides, making the widest arc possible.
- Do 5 Rowings.

TIP! Sit on a pillow to make it easier to stretch your legs and lengthen your spine.

SIDE KICKS FRONT/BACK

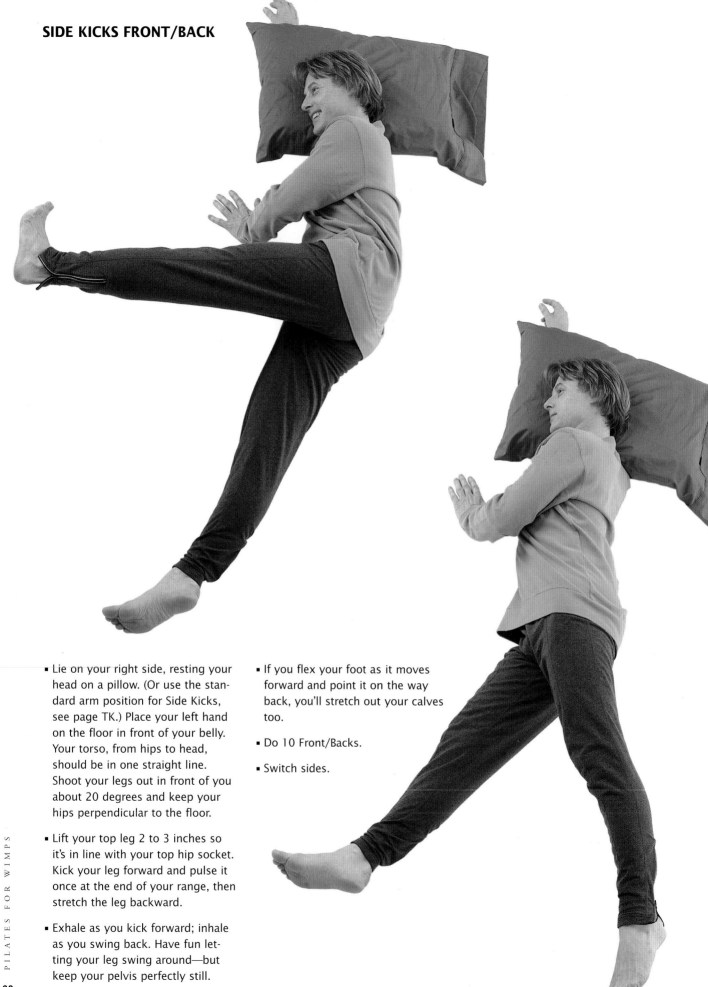

- Lie on your right side, resting your head on a pillow. (Or use the standard arm position for Side Kicks, see page TK.) Place your left hand on the floor in front of your belly. Your torso, from hips to head, should be in one straight line. Shoot your legs out in front of you about 20 degrees and keep your hips perpendicular to the floor.

- Lift your top leg 2 to 3 inches so it's in line with your top hip socket. Kick your leg forward and pulse it once at the end of your range, then stretch the leg backward.

- Exhale as you kick forward; inhale as you swing back. Have fun letting your leg swing around—but keep your pelvis perfectly still.

- If you flex your foot as it moves forward and point it on the way back, you'll stretch out your calves too.

- Do 10 Front/Backs.

- Switch sides.

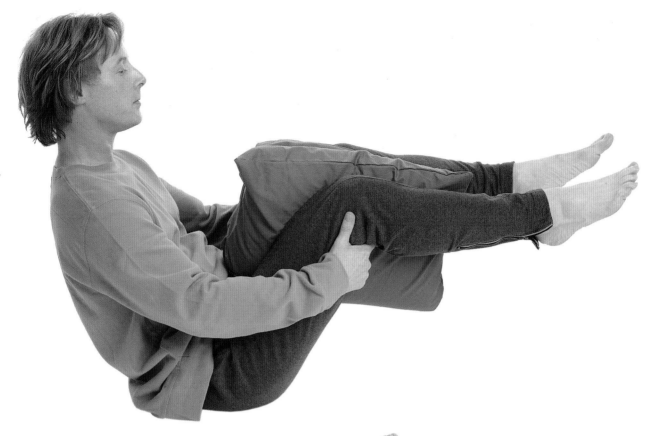

THE LAZY PERSON'S OPEN LEG ROCKER

- Nine times out of ten, people giggle when they do this for the first time, so it must be a mood-lifter!

- Sitting with your legs bent, place a pillow between your knees. (Or you can do without the pillow.) Hold on to the backs of your knees, draw your navel toward your spine, and make a round shape with your body. You should be balancing just behind your tailbone.

- Inhale and roll back to your shoulders. Exhale and rock forward to balance again.

- Do 10 Rockers.

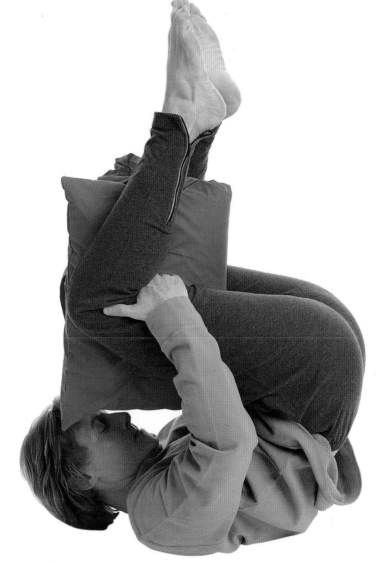

Note: *A more challenging version of this exercise appears in "Bonus Points!" (see page TK).*

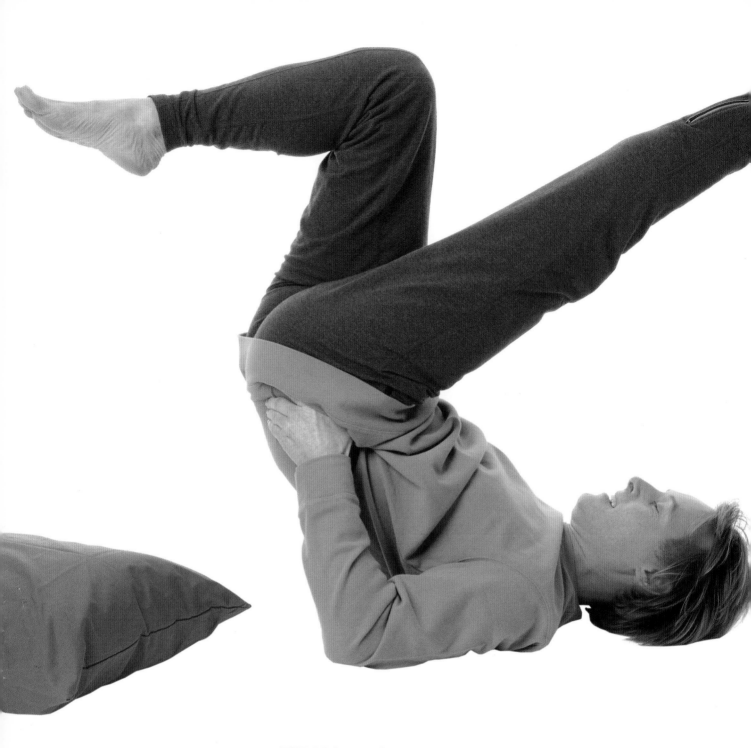

THE UPSIDE DOWN BICYCLE

- Lying on your back, lift your hips in the air and support them with your hands. Your weight should be on your shoulders, not your head.

- Slowly pedal your feet as if you are riding a bicycle. Inhale as one leg extends; exhale as the other extends.

- Pedal 10 times (5 times per side), then reverse directions and pedal 10 times.

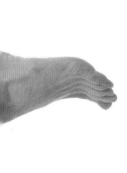

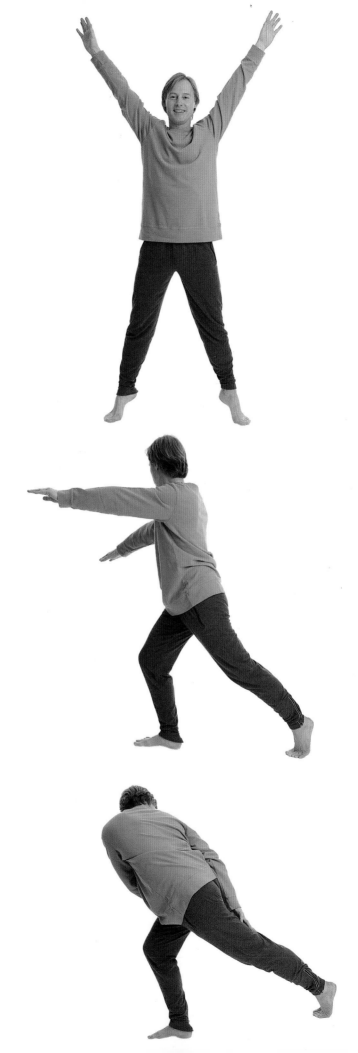

THE STANDING PRETZEL TWIST

- Stand on your toes, arms and legs spread so that you're making an X with your body.

- Twist to your right and bend your right knee. Shift your weight to that leg and try to reach all the way around to grab your left leg with both hands. (Your right heel will come down to the floor as you twist.) Then untwist to form the X again.

- Exhale as you twist; inhale as you untwist.

- Repeat, twisting to the left.

- Do 6 Pretzel Twists (3 on each side).

TIP! If you have difficulty balancing in the X position, pick a spot on the wall to look at. This will often steady you. If it's still too hard, leave your heels on the floor instead of standing on your toes.

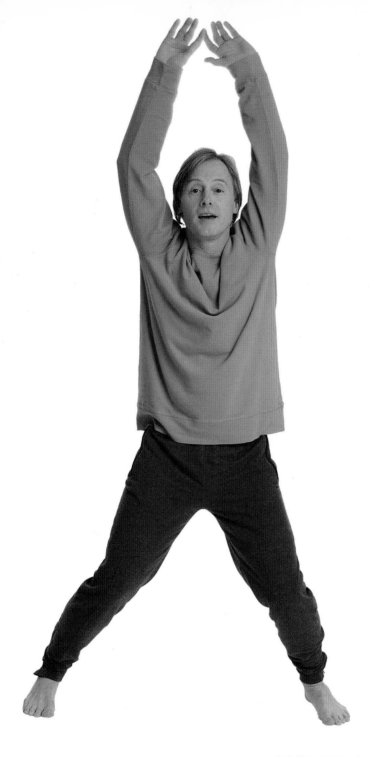

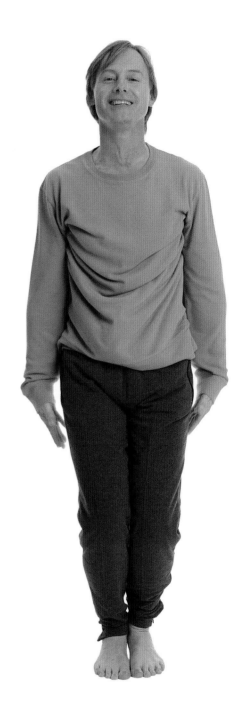

GOOD OLD OLD-FASHIONED
JUMPING JACKS

- Your elementary school gym teacher wasn't totally off. Jumping Jacks are great cardiovascular exercise because, unlike running, they are low-impact (your weight is always distributed between two legs) and you use the arms (which helps stimulate the lungs).

- I recommend doing 50 Jumping Jacks, but go ahead and do more, if you like. They're fun.

TV Exercises

I don't know if Joe would approve of performing your primary exercise program in front of the television, so these are extra exercises that you can squeeze in while you watch TV. This would have him admiring you for your hearty dedication to your personal fitness regime. The exercises are performed sitting down, but that doesn't necessarily mean they are easy! The movements are going to challenge your erector spinae, so it will be difficult to keep a long and elegant posture, especially during the leg lifts. Try not to shrink in height during any of the moves. In fact, try growing an inch or two.

Starting position for TV Exercises: For all the following movements you should be sitting tall, at the edge of your seat (literally), feet flat on the floor, knees and toes pointing forward and hip-width apart.

THIGH LIFT

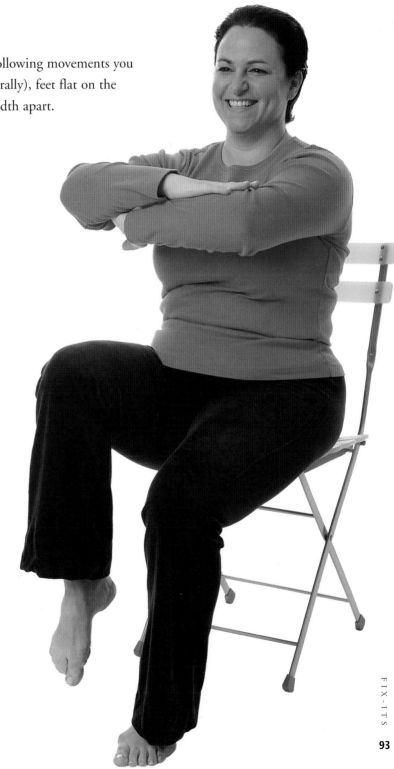

- Fold your arms "genie style" and, trying your hardest to keep your spine in a lengthened position, lift one thigh up. Let the lower portion of your leg dangle loosely toward the floor. Remember to stay tall. Hold for 3 counts.

- Lower your leg and lift it right back up again for 3 counts. Breathe naturally.

- Repeat 5 times.

- Do the same thing on the other side.

TIP! If one side is weaker, start with that leg first, switch to the other leg, then repeat the lifts one more time on the weaker side.

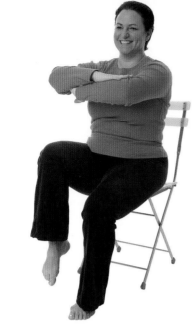

THIGH LIFT WITH HAMSTRING STRETCH

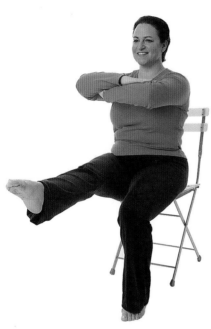

- This one's a little trickier. From the same starting position as before, lift your thigh and try to extend your leg without sinking in height or letting your thigh drop. Hold for 3 counts. Breathe naturally.

- Bend your knee and put your leg back down.

- Don't forget about pulling your belly in and up to support your lower back.

- Do 10 lifts (5 on each side).

Note: *The following exercises are also found on page TK in the standing position. They can be done with or without small weights.*

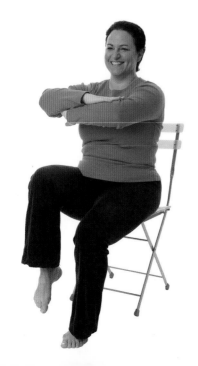

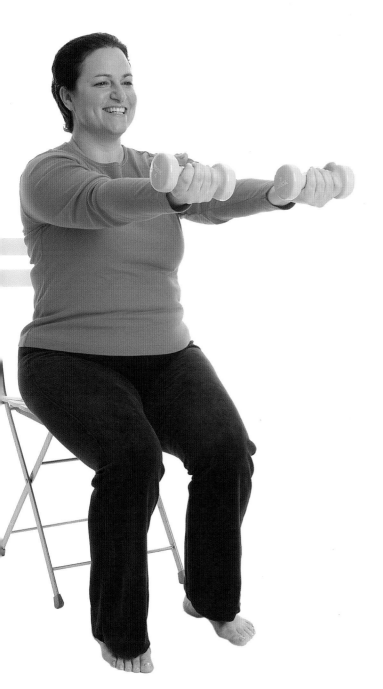
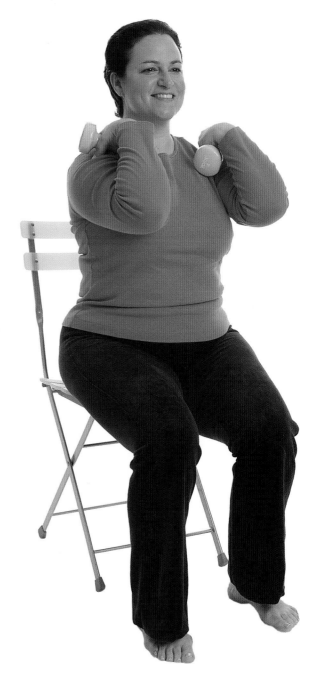

BICEPS CURL FRONT

- Either with or without light weights, raise your arms straight in front of you so they're parallel to the floor, palms up. Bring your hands to touch your shoulders and stretch them back out, with resistance. Exhale as you curl; inhale as you extend.

- Don't drop your elbows. Pretend there's water just below your arms and you don't want your elbows to get wet.

- Do 10 curls.

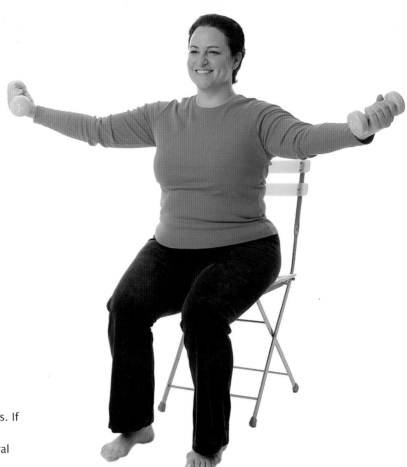

BICEPS CURL SIDE

- Take your arms out to the sides. If you look straight ahead, they should still be in your peripheral vision.

- Curl and uncurl as for Biceps Curl Front. Exhale bringing the arms in; inhale pressing them out.

- Remember—no wet elbows, neck and shoulders relaxed. Are you still pulling your belly button to your spine?

- Do 10 curls.

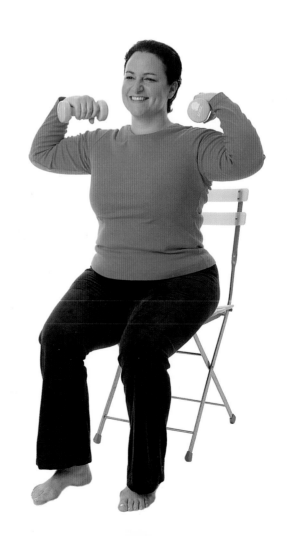

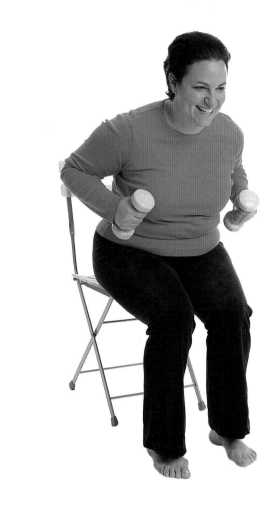

CHICKEN WINGS LEANING FORWARD

- Lean forward, making a diagonal line from your head to your tail-bone. This helps to strengthen the muscles in your back.

- Either holding weights or making fists, point your elbows back and bring your fists up by your shoulders. Press your arms behind you by moving only from the elbows down.

- Exhale as you press back, inhale as you bend.

- Do 10 Chicken Wings.

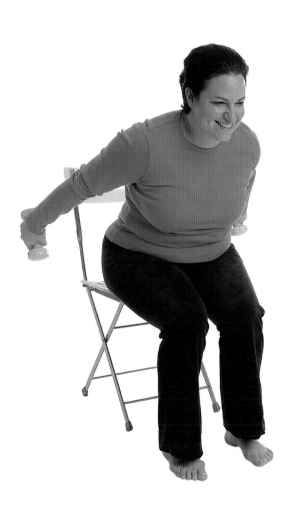

The No-Time-to-Work-Out Workout

Our lives are so jam-packed that we have trouble squeezing the most enjoyable things into them. Thank goodness there's a trend toward fitness—maybe it will bump exercise up a notch or two on your to-do list. This series can be integrated into your day as naturally as brushing your teeth. You'll be using a towel as a prop, so I recommend fitting the moves in right before your shower. I threw in a couple of "toweling off" exercises for afterward, too. The whole thing will take four minutes, once you've learned the movements. With the pleasant buzz you get between the exercise and the shower, you might not need coffee!

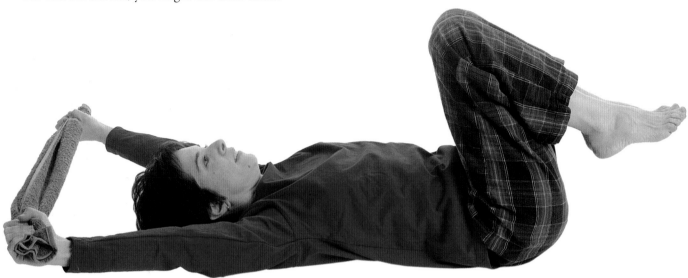

TICK-TOCK WITH ARMS OVERHEAD

- Lie on your back, holding your towel with hands shoulder-width apart. Reach your arms overhead, keeping your ribs and back pressing the floor. Bend your knees in to your chest.

- Slowly tilt your knees over to the right and let your left hip come off

the floor ever so slightly. Then roll back through the center and take your knees to the left.

- Exhale when you "tick" and "tock"; inhale when you return to center.

- Do 8 Tick-Tocks.

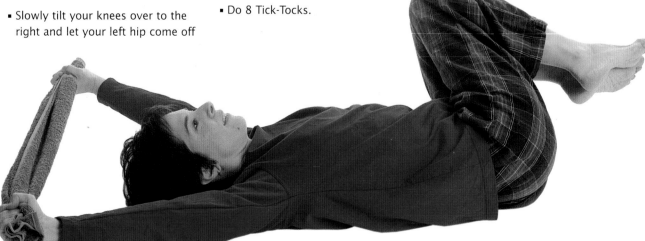

THE HUNDRED WITH TOWEL

- Reach your towel under your legs as you hold them off the floor. It's your choice—extend the legs for more of a challenge; bend the knees to take it easier.

- Lift your head and shoulders off the floor, then pump the towel up and down, breathing in for 5 pumps and exhaling for 5 pumps. Keep your navel actively pulling down to the floor.

- Do this for 10 full, luscious breaths and feel how it energizes you.

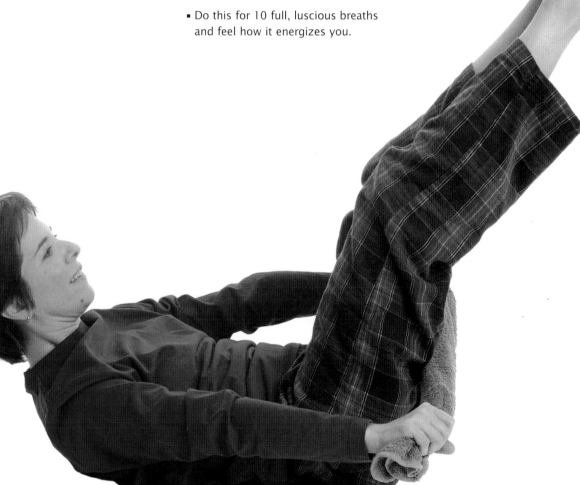

LEG CIRCLES WITH STRETCH

- This is the familiar Leg Circles from page TK with the added help of the towel.

- Lie on your back with your legs bent, feet flat on the floor. Stretch your right leg toward the ceiling. Hook your towel around it wherever feels good—closer to the body will be easier, closer to the foot will be harder. Give the leg 3 gentle stretches by pulling on the towel.

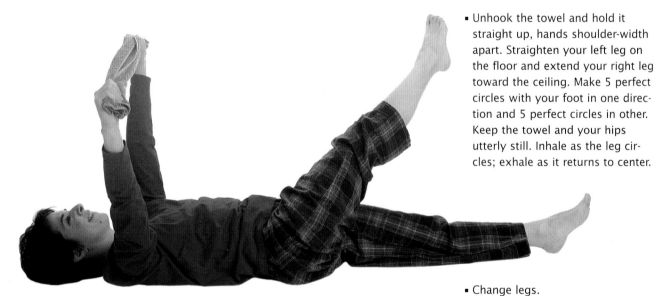

- Unhook the towel and hold it straight up, hands shoulder-width apart. Straighten your left leg on the floor and extend your right leg toward the ceiling. Make 5 perfect circles with your foot in one direction and 5 perfect circles in other. Keep the towel and your hips utterly still. Inhale as the leg circles; exhale as it returns to center.

- Change legs.

TIP! Keep your stabilizing leg bent if you are having trouble keeping your body still.

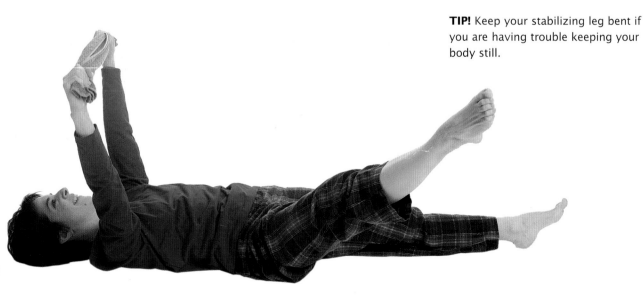

ROLLING LIKE A BALL WITH ARMS EXTENDED

- This is pretty much the same Rolling Like a Ball you saw in Instant Pilates (see page TK).

- Lying on your back, bring your knees to your chest and reach the towel in front of your ankles. Lift your head and shoulders off the floor.

- Make your body into a tight little ball, then get some momentum going and rock yourself up to a balance.

- Rock back to your shoulders (not as far as your head!) and forward so you're sitting again. Inhale as you go back; exhale as you come up.

- Try to keep the curve in your back strong as you support it with your abdominals.

- Do 5 rolls.

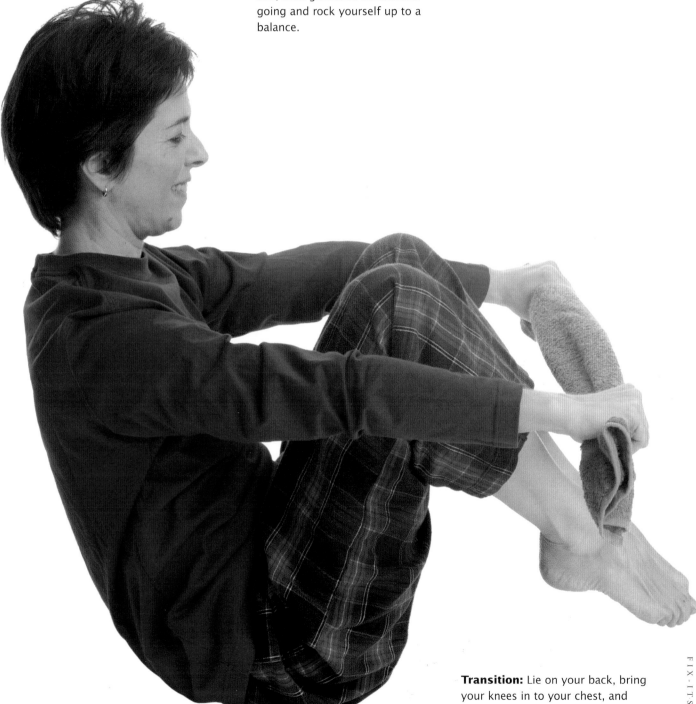

Transition: Lie on your back, bring your knees in to your chest, and reach the towel toward the ceiling.

SINGLE LEG STRETCH WITH TOWEL

- Lift your head and shoulders off the floor. Pull one knee up toward the towel and stretch the opposite leg out in line with your belly button. Change legs.

- Inhale as one knee comes in; exhale for the other.

- Do 10 repetitions (5 times on each side).

TIP! Angling your extended leg more toward the ceiling will make this easier.

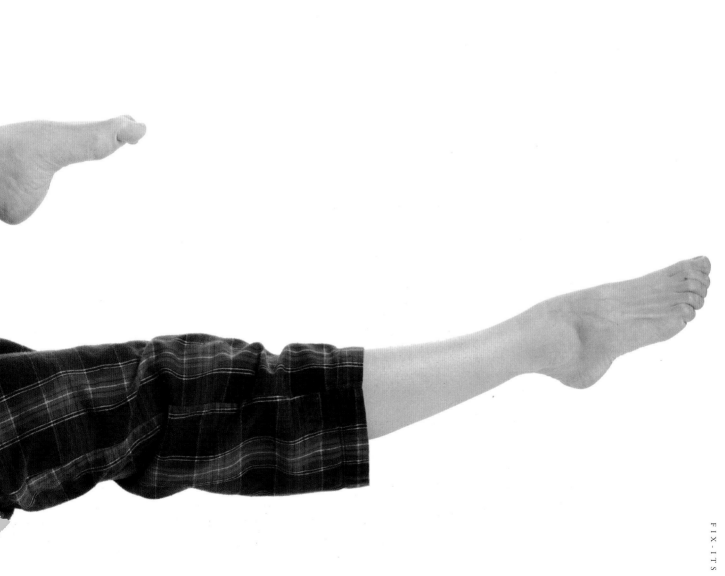

DOUBLE LEG STRETCH WITH TOWEL

- Keep your head and shoulders up from the previous exercise, if you can handle it. Bend both knees under the towel and reach the towel toward your ankles.

- Inhale and extend your legs out to 45 degrees while you stretch the towel overhead. Exhale, bending the knees and reaching the towel toward your ankles again.

- Do 5 stretches.

TIP! Reaching your legs and arms toward the ceiling will make this easier. (Or, if you're feeling ambitious, lower them closer to the floor to make it harder.)

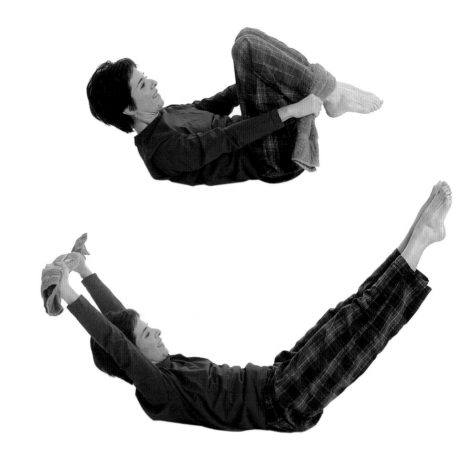

SINGLE STRAIGHT-LEG STRETCH WITH TOWEL

- With head and shoulders still up (if you can do this, you're getting really tough!), stretch the towel toward the ceiling. Tap the towel 2 times with one leg, while the other leg stretches out into space, then switch.

- Your legs should "scissor" past one another. Inhale as you tap with one leg; exhale as you do the other.

- Do 10 stretches (5 times on each side).

NOTE: *The degree to which you spread your legs (and how upright you hold the towel) depends on your flexibility. Most people can't go wider than 90 degrees without screwing up the alignment of the hips. Keep it simple and focus on the stretch of the top leg.*

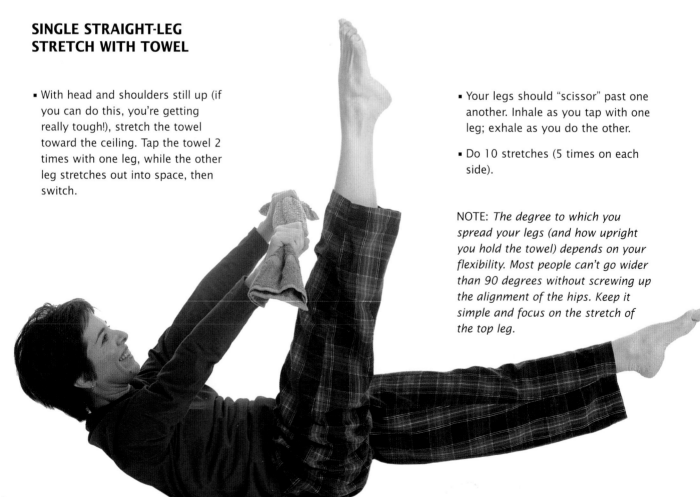

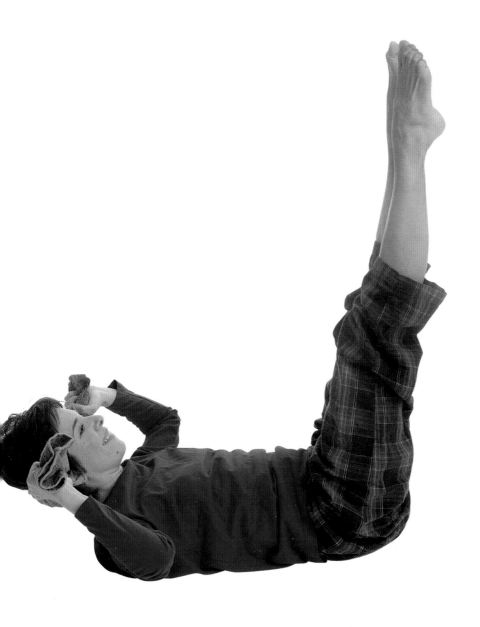

DOUBLE STRAIGHT-LEG STRETCH

- Place the towel around the back of your head to support it. Stretch your legs to the ceiling as straight as possible, then inhale and lower them as much as you can without feeling any strain on your back. (For some of you, this might be an inch; more advanced Pilates practicers might touch the floor.) Exhale to bring the legs back up.

- Keep your legs very active. Dead weight in the legs will be impossible to control and support.

- Do 5 stretches.

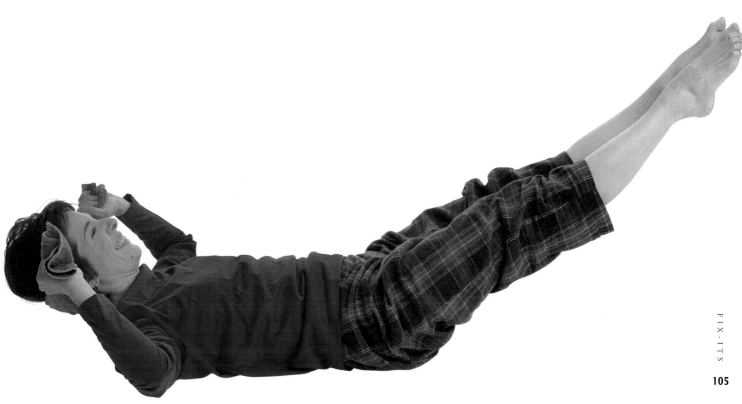

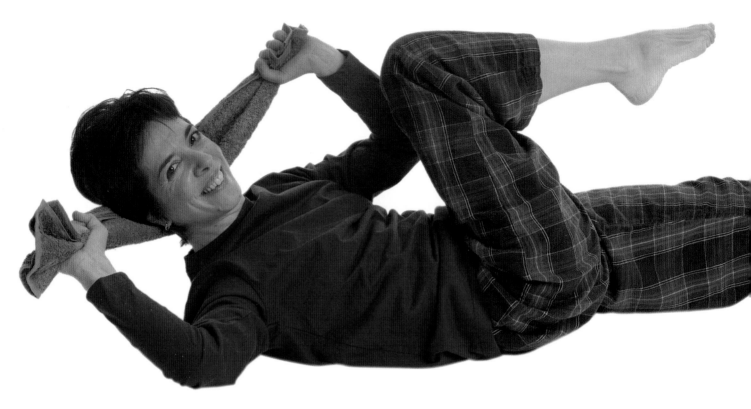

CRISS-CROSS WITH TOWEL

- Keep the towel behind your head to support it. Bring one knee in to touch your opposite elbow. At the same time, extend the other leg in line with your center. Twist to reverse the position.

- Inhale facing one direction; exhale facing the other.

- Do 10 Criss-Crosses (5 on each side).

SPINE STRETCH WITH TOWEL

- Sit tall with your legs in a V position and your towel reaching toward the ceiling.

- Exhaling, round your spine, reach your hands toward your feet, and stretch out through your heels. Pull your tummy toward the back of the room. If you want to, gently pull on the towel to help you stretch.

- Inhale as you roll back up, stacking the bones of the spine one on top of the other, until you return to the starting position.

- Do 5 stretches.

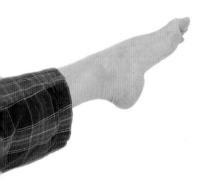

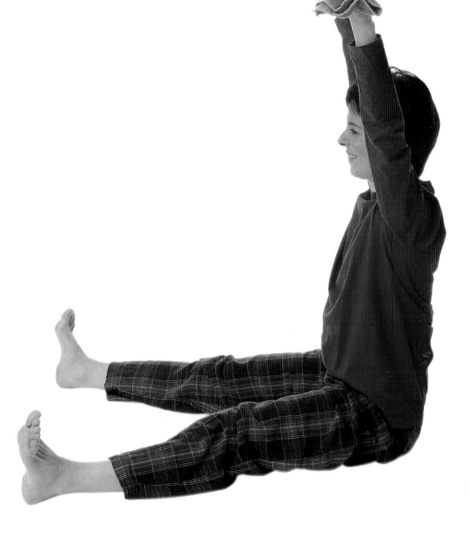

TIP! If your hamstrings are supertight, perform this exercise with the knees bent. When you're in the stretch, push your feet into your towel to increase your hamstring flexibility. For extra help, sit on a pillow as you bend.

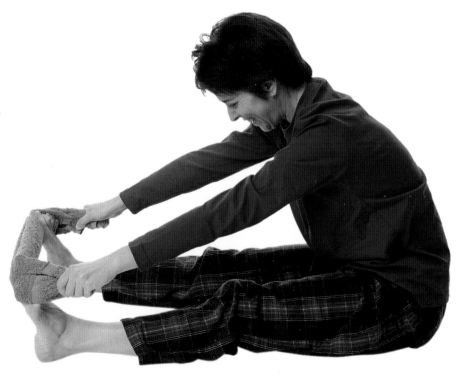

EXTRAS FOR TOWELING OFF

Why have a plain old shower when you can have a shower with whipped cream, hot fudge, and a cherry on top? Sure, a shower is always rejuvenating, but the following add-ons make it feel like a spa treatment. Joe was even mindful of his bathing regimen: He recommended starting with hot water, then gradually decreasing the temperature to cold before you step out. He also believed that it wasn't soap that made you clean but a using good brush to remove dead skin and open the pores—a brush without a handle so you had to stretch and twist to reach everything. Add the following stretches to any bathing ritual for an extra treat.

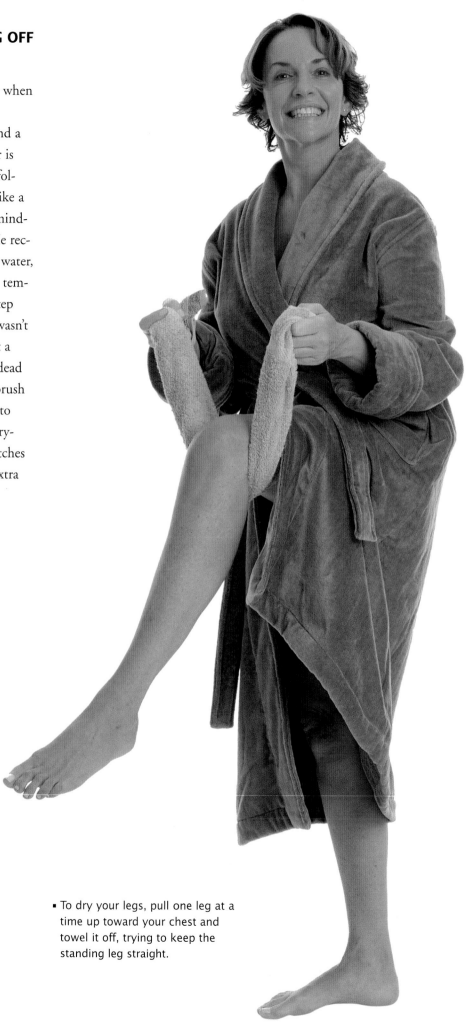

- To dry your legs, pull one leg at a time up toward your chest and towel it off, trying to keep the standing leg straight.

- Place one foot in front of the other and run your towel down the front leg. Try to keep your legs straight. Switch.

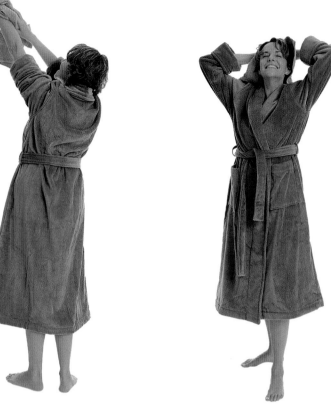

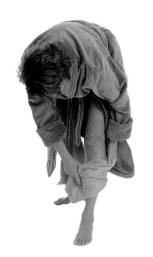

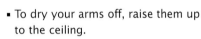

- To dry your arms off, raise them up to the ceiling.

- When drying your head, spend a good 20 seconds (if not more!) massaging your scalp.

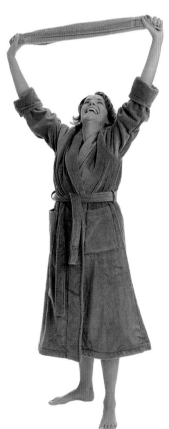

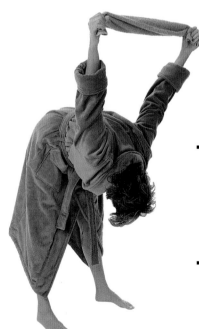

- And now the big finish: Hold the towel behind your back. Your hands could be anywhere from 3 feet apart (easiest) to touching (pretty hard!). Experiment to see what feels best to you.

- Open your legs about 2 feet apart. Exhale and bow forward while lifting your arms toward the ceiling. You deserve to take a bow for putting exercise into your busy day!

- When you're done drying off, hold your towel in both hands, with your arms slightly wider than shoulder-width apart. Stretch your arms straight up and maybe even a little behind you.

The Battle Against Stress and Fatigue

Even though stress and fatigue seem like very different enemies, they have similar effects. Both of them lower the immune system's response, zap vital energy, and tempt you to reach for a potentially damaging quick fix, such as alcohol or caffeine, which just makes everything worse. Luckily, stress and fatigue are also wiped out by similar strategic maneuvers. To conquer these two bad boys, you need rest (both physical and mental), deep breathing, and a little pick-me-up. Think of the following menu as a constructive rest time, a way to decompress and recharge.

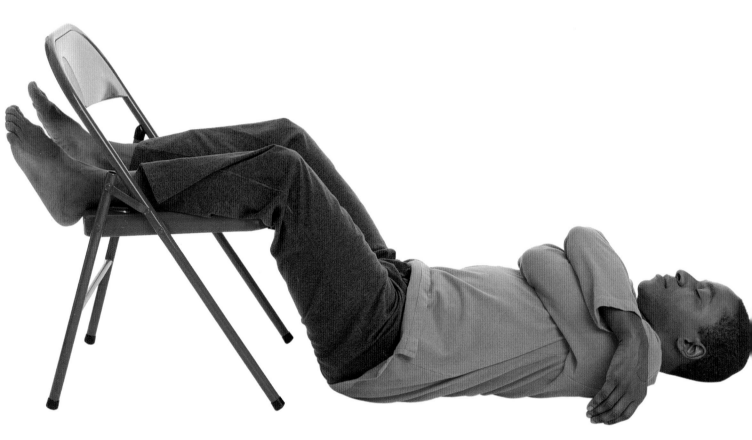

THE CONSTRUCTIVE REST POSITION

- This position is designed to allow your body to fall into its natural alignment without muscular exertion. Gravity does all the work. Lie on your back with your lower legs resting on a chair. Fold your arms across your chest or belly.

- Allow your body to give in to gravity and stay there as long as you like. As much as 20 minutes is fine—in fact, it's recommended.

- Focus on your breathing. If your mind keeps attaching to a nagging thought, give your breath a color. For example, concentrate on inhaling blue and exhaling gold.

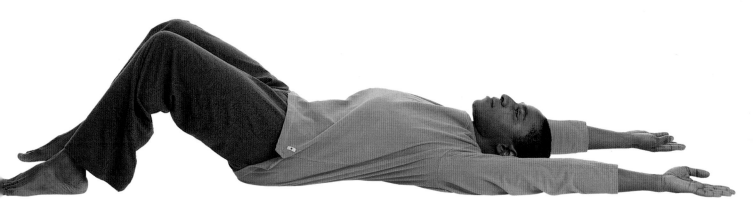

THE BREATHING

- Place your feet on the floor, knees bent and feet hip-width apart, arms stretched overhead. Inhale, lifting your hips and bringing your arms down until they're parallel to your thighs. Hold your breath in this position for 5 counts.

- Exhale and roll back down bone by bone, stretching your arms overhead again. Be sure to keep your knees pointing straight ahead the entire time.

- Do 5 Breathings.

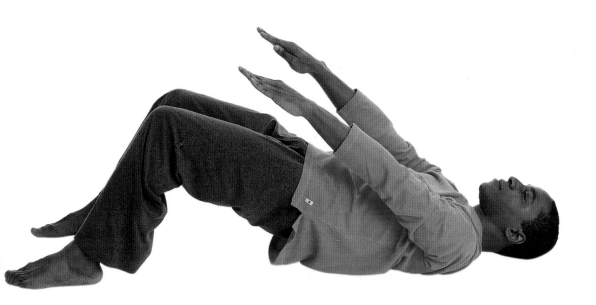

- This is just like the sitting-down version of the Saw that you'll learn in "Bonus Points!" (see page TK), but gravity changes the stretch.

- Stand with your legs 2 to 3 feet apart and your arms reaching out to the sides. Exhale, bending over and extending your right pinky finger toward your left pinky toe. Inhale to return to standing tall.

- Repeat, twisting in the opposition direction.

- Do 6 Saws, alternating sides.

CRISS-CROSS

- Place your hands behind your head and lift your head and shoulders off the floor. Stretch your left leg to 45 degrees and bend your right knee into the chest.

- Keeping your pelvis completely still, twist to touch your left elbow to your right knee. Change to do the other side. Inhale in one direction; exhale in the other.

- Do 10 Criss-Crosses, alternating sides.

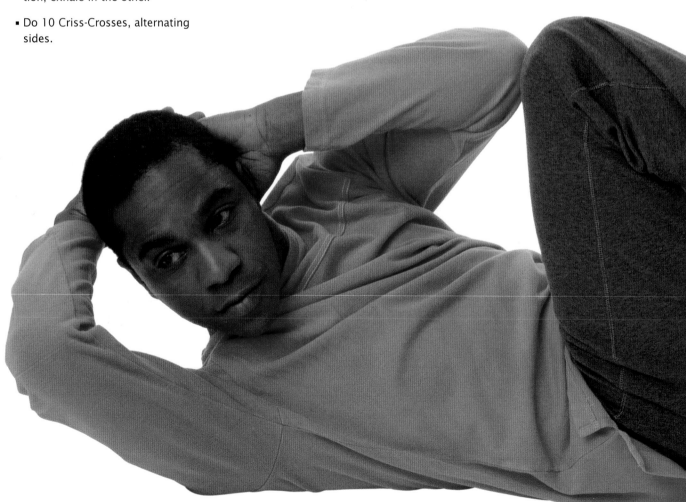

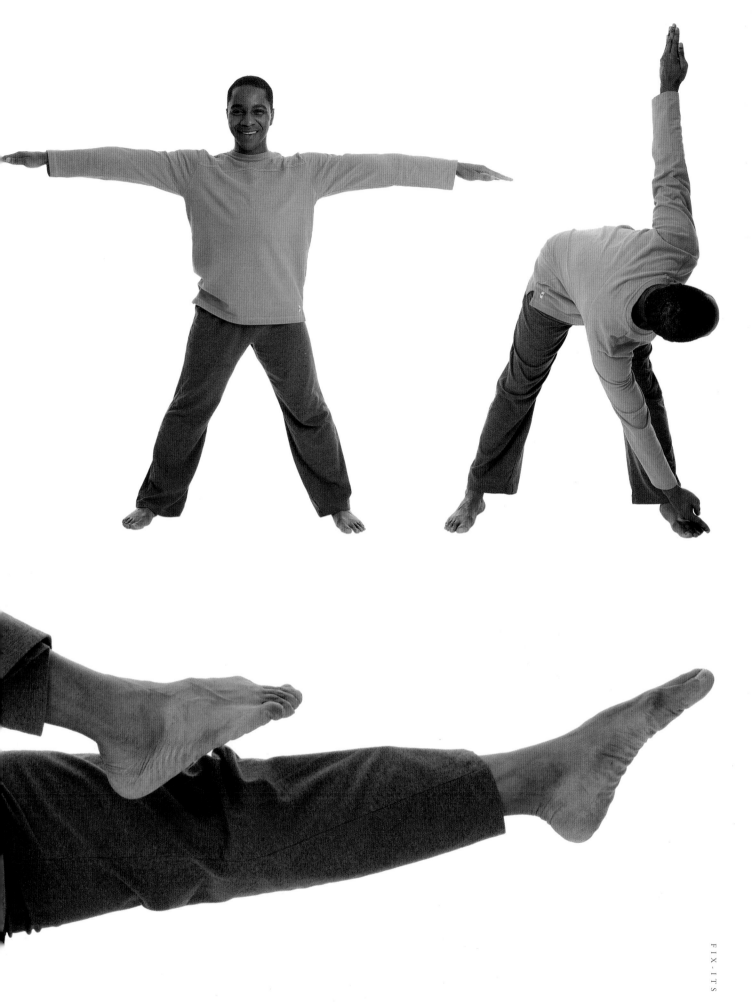

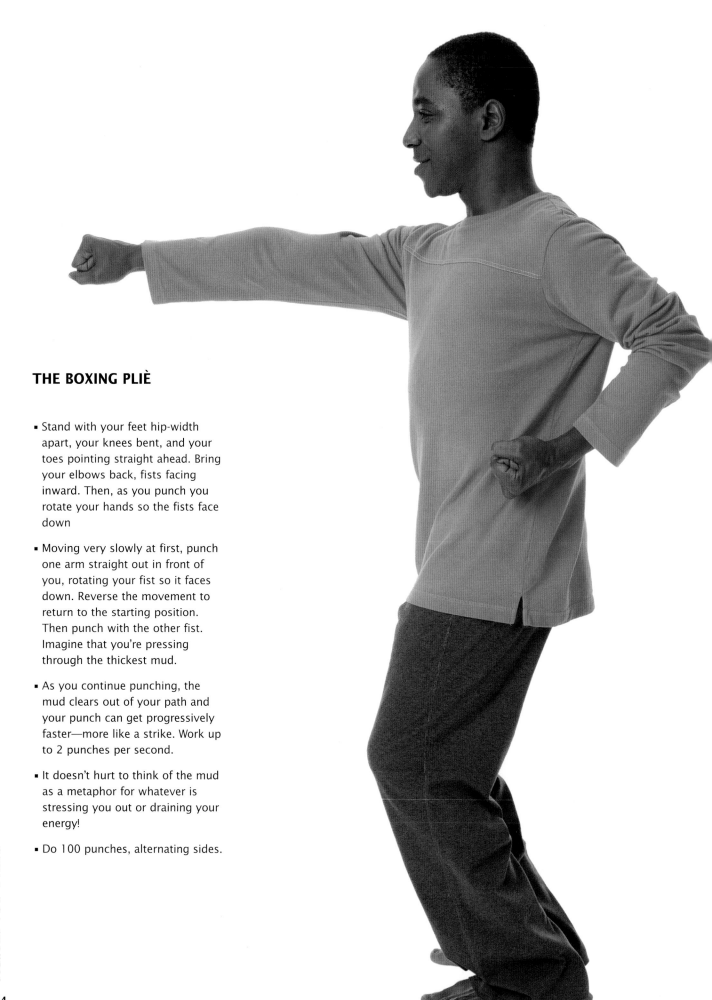

THE BOXING PLIÈ

- Stand with your feet hip-width apart, your knees bent, and your toes pointing straight ahead. Bring your elbows back, fists facing inward. Then, as you punch you rotate your hands so the fists face down

- Moving very slowly at first, punch one arm straight out in front of you, rotating your fist so it faces down. Reverse the movement to return to the starting position. Then punch with the other fist. Imagine that you're pressing through the thickest mud.

- As you continue punching, the mud clears out of your path and your punch can get progressively faster—more like a strike. Work up to 2 punches per second.

- It doesn't hurt to think of the mud as a metaphor for whatever is stressing you out or draining your energy!

- Do 100 punches, alternating sides.

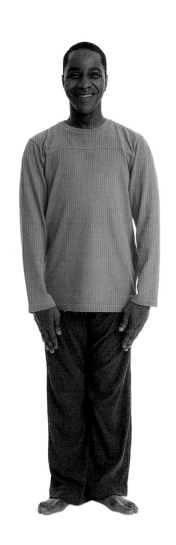

SIDE SPLITS STANDING

- Stand with your arms resting at your sides and your heels together so that your feet form a V.

- Take a giant step to the side with your left leg—a nice, juicy lunge. At the same time, raise your arms until they're parallel to the floor. Then, in one swift move, return to the starting position.

- Lunge to the right and return to standing.

- Follow the timing of your breathing. Exhale for the lunge; inhale on the way back.

- Do 10 Side Splits, alternating sides.

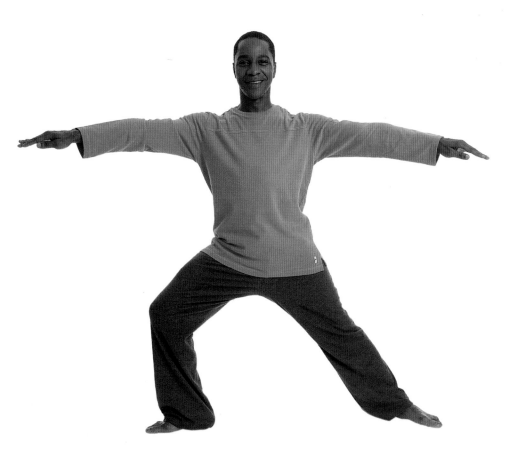

The exercises you are about to see are indeed a full, intense, and classic Mat routine. Don't be afraid! Most of them are ones you've already mastered, with a modification or two to amp 'em up. You can do one of the extra challenges or both, depending on what feels best to you. There are a few brand-new feats to accomplish too. Those are presented with more explanation to help you along. These exercises can be incredibly challenging and really fun to do. I recommend perusing the photos in this section before doing anything you haven't done before. When you're up for it, pick one or two exercises that look intriguing. Add them to your personal Mat routine little by little. Pilates is exercise for a lifetime, so there's no rush to get it all in right this second.

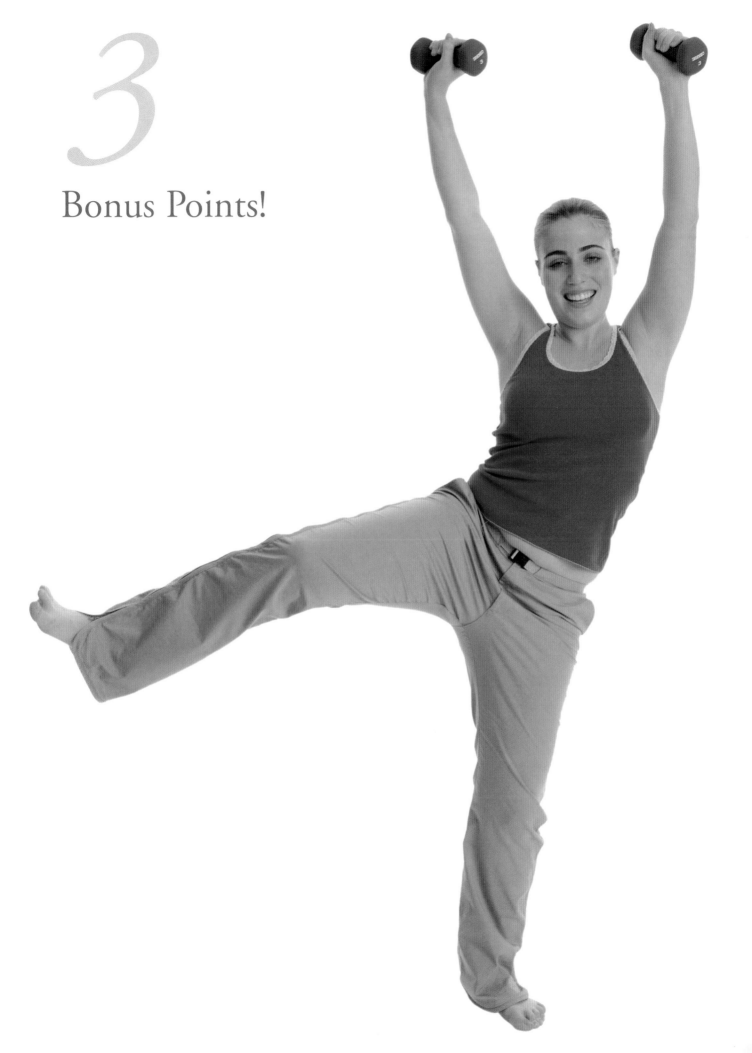

3

Bonus Points!

Before you proceed into this new and exciting territory of higher-level exercises, there are a few things you should have securely stowed in your body and mind:

1. A firm understanding of the powerhouse and what it means to initiate from, and stabilize with, this area.

2. No major injuries. Pilates can work out your kinks, but if you're somewhat fragile at the moment, get professional advice first.

3. A solid memory of the Mat routine given in "Instant Pilates." If you're constantly flipping pages, you're not getting the benefits. Your flow, concentration, and breathing will be constantly disrupted.

4. Keen awareness of your body. If you've been doing the Mat routine for the appropriate amount of time, you understand exactly what I mean here. Your body has undoubtedly gotten better at communicating what it needs and can handle. Use that awareness to choose new exercises that suit *you*.

5. Look for this to see completely new stuff to try.

Beyond Instant Pilates
The Advanced Routine

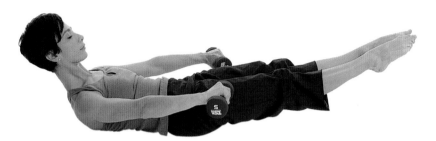

THE HUNDRED

- Take your legs lower toward the floor.

- Hold light weights as you pump your arms.

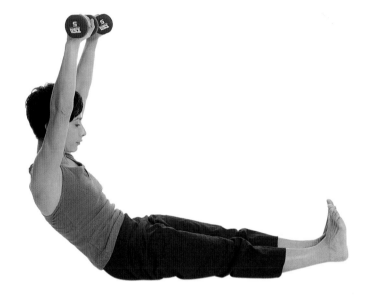

THE ROLL-UP

- Keep your upper arms by your ears the whole time.

- Hold light weights.

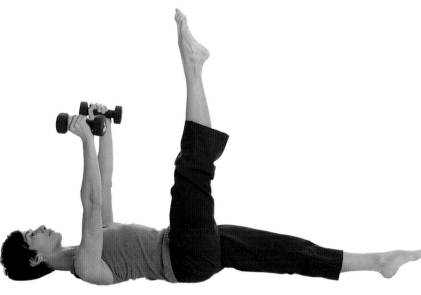

LEG CIRCLES

- Make the circles bigger.

- Hold your weights toward the ceiling and keep them perfectly still.

ROLLING LIKE A BALL

- Place your hands on opposite ankles, making a tighter ball.

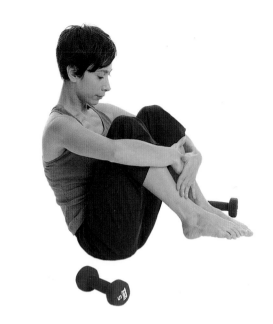

SINGLE LEG STRETCH

- Hold light weights and reach your arms toward the ceiling instead of holding your leg with your hands.

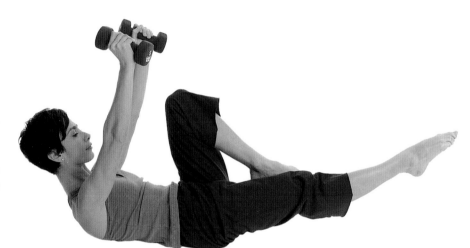

DOUBLE LEG STRETCH

- Try it with your legs lower.
- Hold light weights.

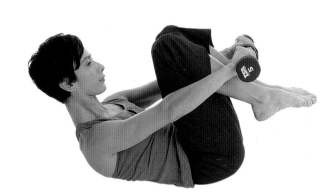

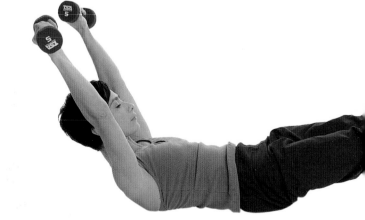

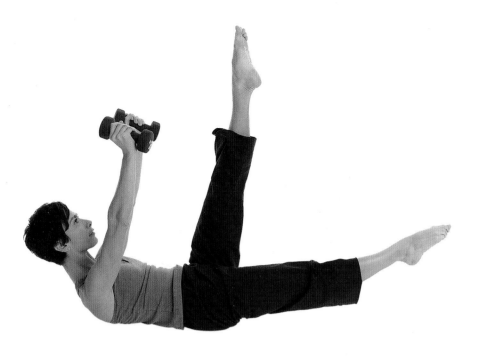

SINGLE STRAIGHT-LEG STRETCH

- Hold light weights and reach your arms toward the ceiling.

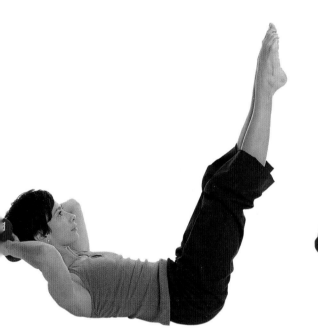

DOUBLE STRAIGHT-LEG STRETCH

- Lower your legs as close to the floor as you can.
- Hold light weights behind your head.

CRISS-CROSS

- Hold light weights behind your head.

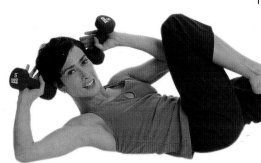

SPINE STRETCH

- Keep your arms by your ears the whole time.

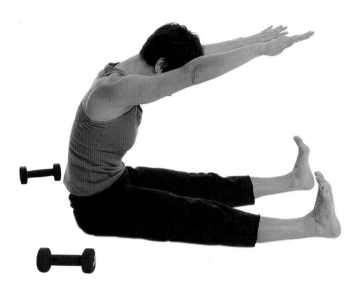

Transition: Bring your feet together as in the Seal (see page 53).

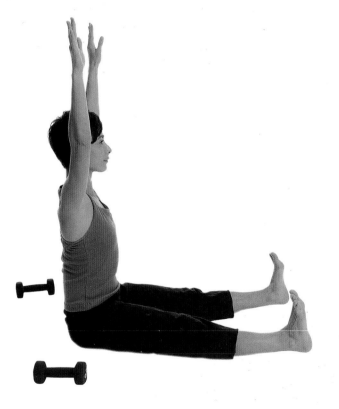

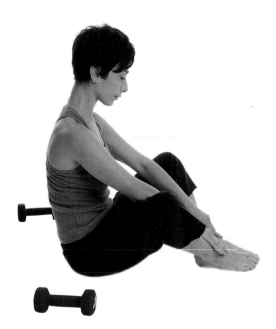

OPEN LEG ROCKER

- Hold the tops of your ankles and stretch both legs into a V position while balancing just behind your tailbone.

- Inhale to rock back to your shoulders, maintaining your position. Exhale to come back to a perfect balance.

- Do 5 Open Leg Rockers.

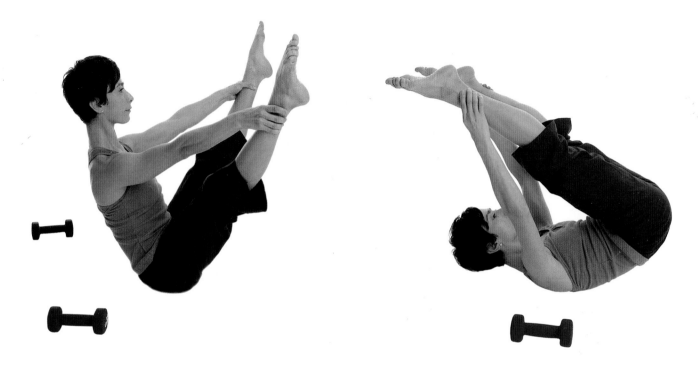

Transition: Bring your feet back to the Seal position and extend your legs to form a V on the floor. Flex your feet.

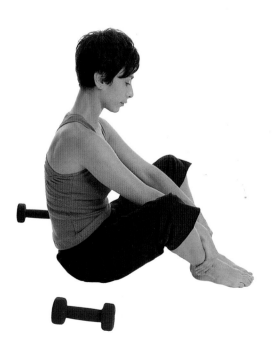

THE SAW

- Master this without weights first—you can add them later.

- Stretch your arms out to the sides and inhale deeply.

- Exhale, twisting your upper body toward your right leg, and reach your left pinky finger past your right pinky toe to "saw off" the toe. Inhale as you come back to the sitting position.

- Reverse the twist and saw off your left pinky toe.

- Keep your pelvis perfectly still so that you use, and stretch, your oblique abdominals.

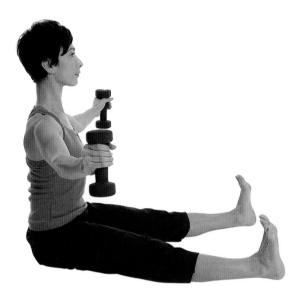

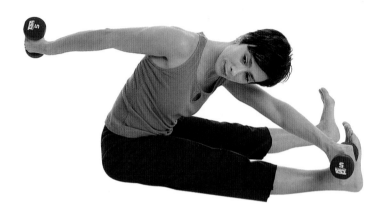

- To challenge your arms a bit more, press the back arm, palm up, toward the ceiling.

- Do 6 Saws (3 on each side).

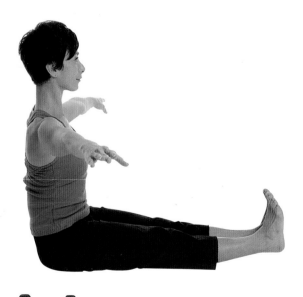

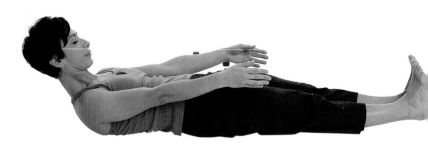

Transition: Bring your legs together, then roll down bone by bone to the floor and turn over onto your tummy.

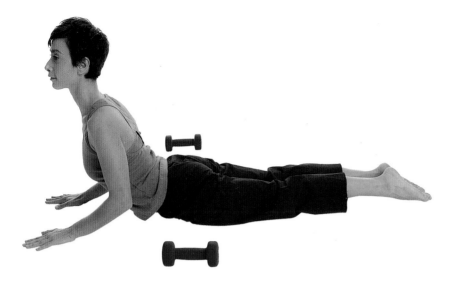

SIMPLE BACK EXTENSION

- Do it with your legs together— don't let them part!

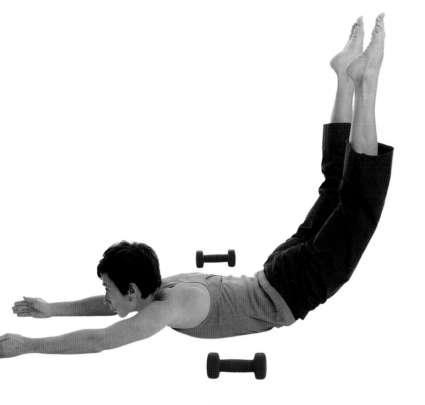

SWAN DIVE

- Press up once more, as in the Simple Back Extension. Imagine that your body is shaped like the runners on a rocking chair.

- Shoot your hands out in front of you and rock your weight forward toward your chest. Keep your legs long and stretched as they rise up, then let the momentum bring them back down as you lift your chest off the floor. Exhale as the chest comes down; inhale as it comes up.

- You must hold the bowed shape throughout your entire body to maintain the momentum and keep your back from taking on too much work—keep thinking of the rocking chair.

- Do 5 Swan Dives.

SINGLE LEG KICK

- Turn your fists to press against each other and aim your elbows out to the sides. Firmly and constantly press into the floor with your forearms.

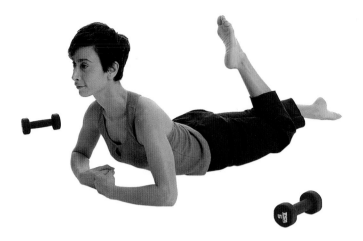

DOUBLE LEG KICK

- Lift your chest off the floor completely.

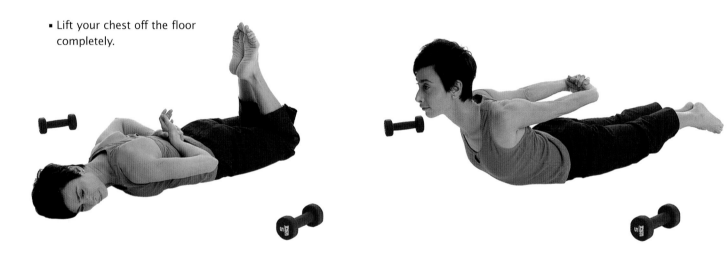

Transition: Take a moment's rest in Child's Pose.

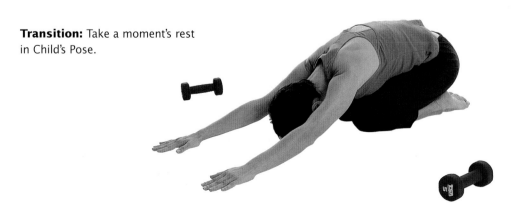

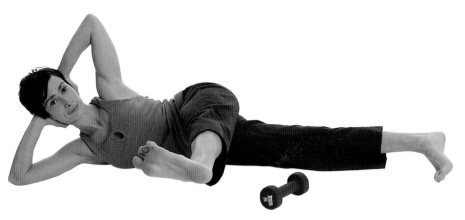

SIDE KICKS FRONT/BACK

▪ Place both hands behind your head so you won't have stabilizing help from your arm. Don't let your hips or shoulders move!

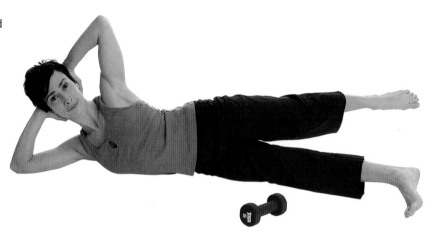

SIDE KICKS UP/DOWN

▪ Keep your hands behind your head. And remember: hips and shoulders completely still.

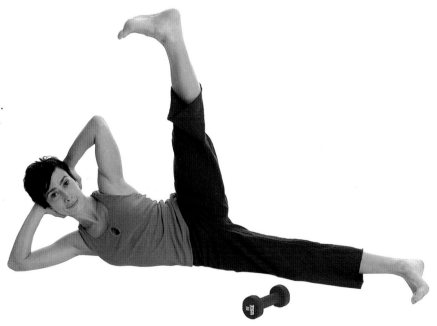

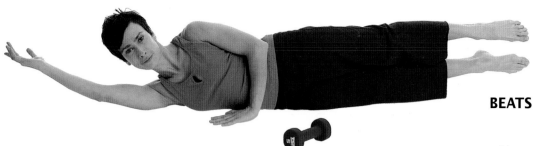

BEATS

- (You can bring your top hand to the floor for support now.) Lift your head and lower arm while you do your beats.

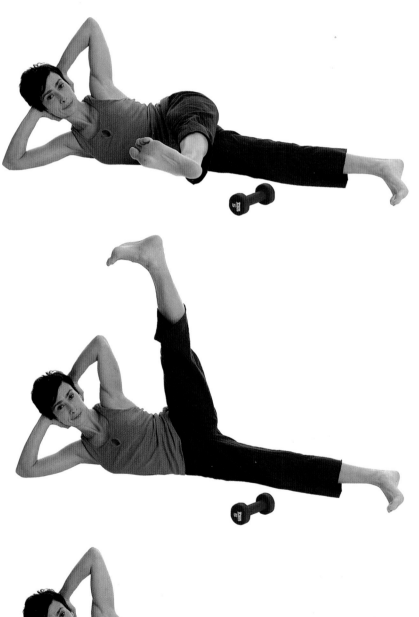

GIANT (EVIL) CIRCLES

- Again, no support hand and keep your torso still. Now, instead of making a circle the size of a bubble, you're going to make one as big as a gymnasium! Reach your leg in front of you as far as you can, then as high as you can to the side, and, finally, as far to the back as possible. (When reaching to the back, think about stretching your leg away from your hips and keeping your lower back long.)

- Inhale as the leg travels to the front and side. Exhale as it moves back and returns to the starting position.

- Do 3 circles in each direction.

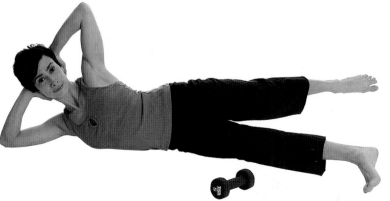

Transition: Repeat all the Side Kicks for the other leg, then roll onto your back.

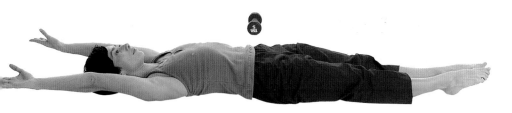

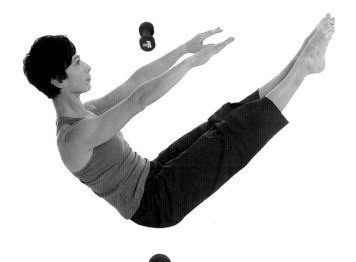

THE TEASER

- Remember to begin your movement by bringing your navel in and up. Instead of bending your legs, keep them straight. At the height of the V, lift your arms, then roll down with control.

- For an even more advanced version, start with your arms stretched over your head as you lie on the floor.

- And to make this super-duper hard, add weights.

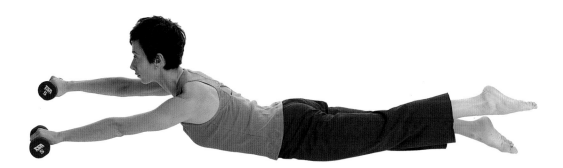

SWIMMING

- Swim with light weights in your hands.

Transition: A moment's rest in Child's Pose.

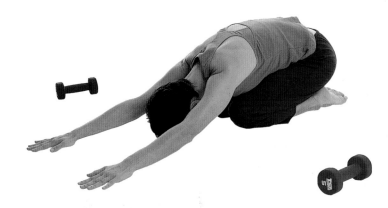

KNEELING SIDE KICKS

- Come to kneeling and then "fall over" onto your right hand, with your fingers facing away from you.

- Place your left hand behind your head and stretch your left leg so it's parallel to the floor. Swing your leg to the front, pulse it once, then stretch it to the back.

- Don't let your leg change in height and keep your supporting arm and entire torso active. Exhale as you kick to the front; inhale as you go back.

- Do 5 kicks and then, in one swift motion, bring your body back to the kneeling position.

- "Fall" to the other side and repeat.

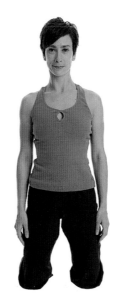

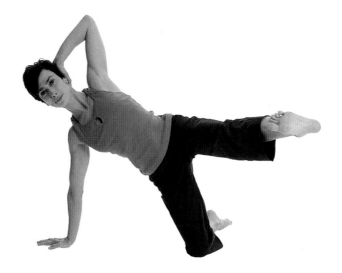

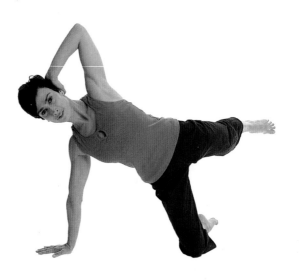

Starting position: From the kneeling position, sit on your left hip. Hold your right ankle with your right hand and stretch your left arm up to the ceiling.

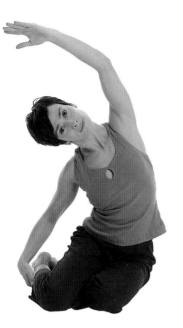

THE MERMAID WITH SIDE BALANCE

- Exhale and bend sideways toward your feet. Inhale to return to the starting position.

- Reach your left hand out to the side and place it on the floor. As you do this, extend your right foot in the opposite direction, placing the bottom of your foot on the floor. Lift your hips and cross your left leg in front of your right leg.

- To really complete the position, stretch your top arm up to the ceiling.

- Come down, lowering first your left leg, then your hips to the floor and bringing your heels toward your bottom again.

- Do 3 Mermaids.

- Switch so your legs are to the other side and repeat.

Transition: Lie face down on the floor.

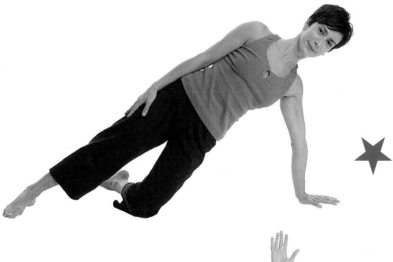

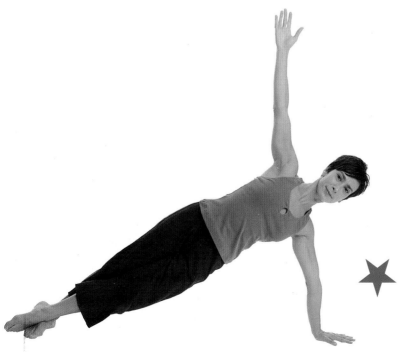

ROCKING

- You've already learned the prep for this one. If you're ready to move on, rock forward and back like a rocking horse. Exhale while rolling toward your chest; inhale while rolling toward your pubic bone.

- Do 5 Rockings.

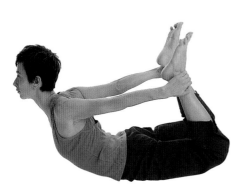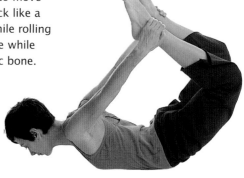

THE SEAL

- Guess what? This one's a gift. . . . The Seal is always the same.

- Do 5 and finish the last one by coming to standing.

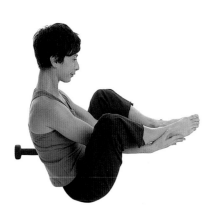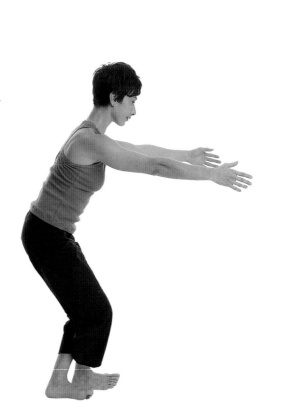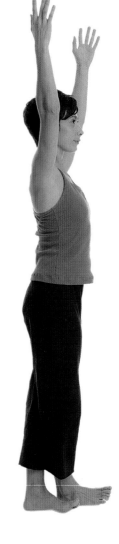

Ta da! You have now added some advanced movements to your repertoire. Feel free to leave it at that or finish with the Arm Series or the Wall. Both are lovely ways to cap off your personal routine. For a more challenging finish, I'm about to give you a Push-Up Series that Romana Kryzanowska used with all the hard-bodied apprentices at Drago's Gym, as well as three new, more-advanced Arm Series exercises.

The Push-Ups

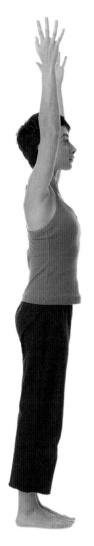

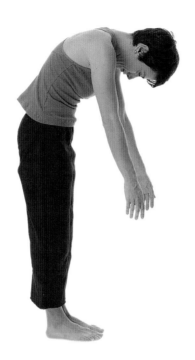

PUSH-UP #1

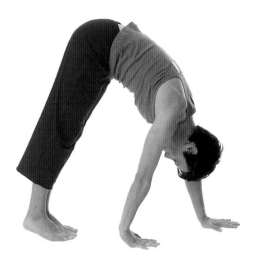

- Start out standing with your feet together, toes facing forward, and arms stretching to the ceiling. Beginning with your head and arms, slowly curl your body toward the floor. Once your hands touch the floor, walk out to a push-up position. Place your hands just wider than shoulder-width apart.

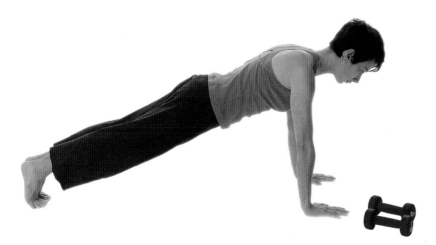

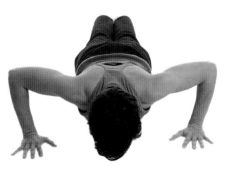

- Now that you're here, you have a lot of leeway. You can do 1 push-up or 20—just be sure to keep your body in a straight line as you bend and straighten your elbows.

Inhale as you lower your body; exhale as you push the floor away.

- When you're finished, walk your hands back and slowly "uncurl" to return to the starting position.

PUSH-UP #2

- Again, starting from standing, slowly curl to the floor and walk your hands out. This time, your hands must be placed directly beneath the shoulders, and when you bend your arms to lower your body, try to get your elbows to touch the seams of your T-shirt. Inhale as you lower and exhale as you push the floor away.

- The focus here is on the triceps, and these push-ups are *much more difficult* to do. Just one of them can be incredibly challenging, so do only what you can without sacrificing your alignment.

- Walk your hands back and uncurl to standing.

PUSH-UP #3

- Same beginning as before, but this time walk out only far enough to make an upside-down V with your body. Lower the crown of your head to the floor as you bend your elbows. Inhale as you lower and exhale as you push the floor away.

- When you've done as many push-ups as you want to, walk your hands back and slowly uncurl.

- After you stretch your arms toward the ceiling, wrap your left arm around your waist to the front and your right arm around to the back and take a bow!

Arm Series Add-Ons

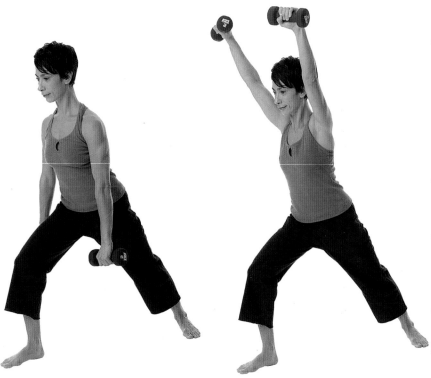

THE LUNGE

- Holding your weights, begin with your feet in a small V. Imagine a line projecting out from your middle toe and take a giant step into a lunge along that line. Pitch your upper body forward to create one long diagonal from your head to your back heel.

- Inhale as you raise your weights forward and up; exhale as you lower them.

- Try to keep your back heel down to stretch the calf, and try to keep your pelvis facing your front foot to stretch the hips properly.

- Lift and lower your arms 10 times, then return to the starting position.

- Repeat for the other leg.

THE BOXING

- Holding your weights, open your legs so they are hip-width apart. Bend your knees, aiming them directly over your toes, and lean forward to make a "tabletop" with your torso—you should be pretty much parallel to the floor from head to tail. It will feel as if you're bending your knees quite a bit.

- Slowly punch your right arm forward while you bring your left arm back. Then, punch your left arm forward and bring your right arm back.

- Be sure not to swing your arms. Move by bending the elbow joints instead. Also, keep your head and tail in one line. People tend to wiggle their butts a little as they do this!

- Inhale as you punch with one arm; exhale for the other.

- Do 10 Boxings (5 on each side).

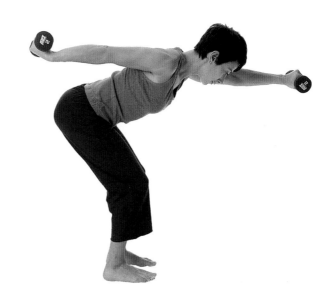

Note: To come upright, first drop your head and hands toward the floor, then roll up, bringing your head up last. Make this your ending for both exercises.

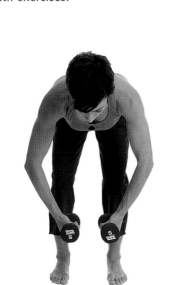

THE BUG

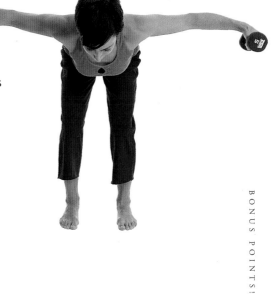

- Starting in the same body position as for the Boxing, round your arms with your weights aiming at the floor. Open your arms to the sides of the room without changing the shape of your elbow joints. In other words, move from your upper arm and take your elbows with you.

- Inhale as you open; exhale as you control down.

- Do 10 Bugs.

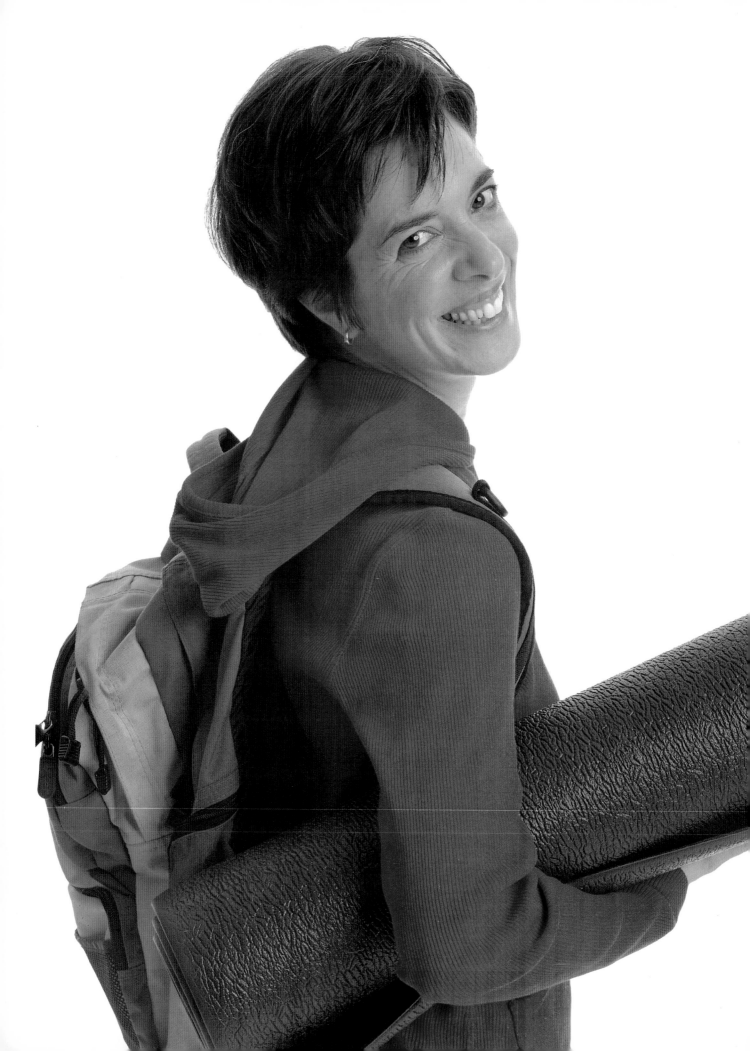

A Final Word

"To exercise or not to exercise?" That is the daily, weekly, perhaps yearly, question. Why is something so natural to the human condition (movement) so aggressively avoided? There are many valid reasons: computers, hectic lifestyles, faster pizza delivery. But I think that even when people try to add exercise to their crammed lives—even *after* they make the effort and get to the class, join the gym, run the mile or two—something negative stops the momentum. It might be the soreness, the awkwardness, or the monotonous movements. Whatever the reason, a bad exercise experience is worse than never having gotten off the couch at all. It's defeating, and in the end people learn to despise exercise.

As you ponder the exercise question, you can't ignore the fact that "to exercise" is the better choice. In some ways, it's the only choice. Sure, there are people out there who avoid unnecessary physical activity at all costs. But they pay the price somewhere down the line. Human beings were undoubtedly meant to move. They undoubtedly get more pleasure out of life when they are fit. And this is not only during our teens and early adulthood. At 40, 50, 60, 70, 80 years old, we need to keep moving for our bodies to function properly and

for our lives to flourish. If our lifestyles don't lend themselves to that physicality, it's up to us to do something about it.

If I sound like I'm professing the tenets of life, well, then, it must be the spirit of Joe. I am completely sympatico with him on this. I've seen it hundreds of times—a life transformed through the Pilates technique. It may sound like quackery now and, chances are, it did back in the 1920s when Joe was starting out. But this "quackery" has helped so many people, from elite dancers to the likes of NBA star Jason Kidd. It tumbled into, and flooded, the mainstream in a relatively short period of time. Why? Because somehow, through an innate gift, a genius who understood the needs of the human body constructed a thorough series of movements and a mental philosophy to meet those needs.

While writing this book, I remained dedicated to Joe Pilates' original intentions. Any modifications were based on current information about the human body and proper alignment. I felt (and always feel) it is my duty to communicate his work with a sense of purity and the utmost respect for his technique. My goal is to teach his work the way it was intended—

with intelligence, precision, flow, and spirit. Its integrity relies on these qualities and the performer's complete physical commitment to the movements. The more you get into it, the more you get out of it, and the more you get out of it, the better you feel. I hope you enjoy the physicality, diversity, challenges, soothing sensations, and positive aftereffects. A strong body, intelligent coordination, and the freedom and pleasure of being limber and agile are all your birthright.

You are holding a better life in your hands. Enjoy.

Index

About the Models

These folks—many of whom are the author's Pilates students—were game and good-natured enough to model for *Pilates for Wimps*. Thanks and kudos to them for their energy, patience, flexibility of schedule, and enthusiastic spirit.

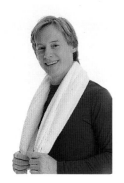

Randy St. Louis has lived since 1982 in Manhattan, where he is the manager of a popular Times Square restaurant. He has been doing Pilates for two years and has found it to be the best exercise to alleviate a longstanding problem with his lower back.

Gabrielle Nakash, when she's not practicing Pilates, is hard at work further developing her sense of style and figuring out new ways to become a superstar. Trained as a chef, she is a self-professed drama queen who prefers eating the food to preparing it—and therefore depends upon Pilates to keep her in shape!

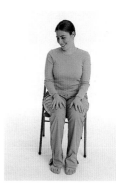

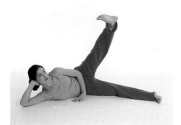

Bianca Craig, originally from British Columbia, Canada, moved to New York to train as an actress. An ex-figure skater, she discovered Pilates while rehabilitating an injury. (Bianca now believes that all figure skaters and hockey players should practice Pilates as part of their off-ice conditioning.) She is a self-proclaimed sugar addict who, these days, relies solely on Pilates to keep her in shape.

Dan Dome is a video editor and musician who lives in New York City. He'd never done Pilates prior to participating in this photo shoot as a favor to a good friend. This was his favorite exercise.

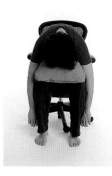

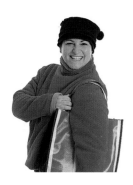

Marla Bloch Kochman works for an international bank as a banking attorney. She lives in Park Slope, Brooklyn, with her three sons and her husband, all of whom can actually pronounce "Pilates" and have done "The Hundred" on more than one occasion at home. Marla has been doing Pilates for five years, and credits the regimen for giving her the mental and physical strength to balance a demanding and chaotic life.

Dayna Bealy reckons she has the tightest hamstrings on the planet. She is photo editor for a large non-profit organization and lives in Brooklyn with her husband and two teenage sons. She has grown a quarter inch in the two years she has been practicing Pilates!

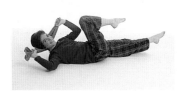

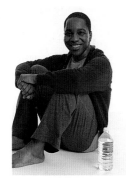

Donald Porter is a dancer and has been studying Pilates for a year and a half. He hopes to someday acquire a certificate to teach Pilates.

Karen Brothers is a former ballet student turned hip-hop dancer turned social worker turned proud mom of daughter Tatia. She is grateful to Pilates for helping her body to catch up with all the other twists and turns in her life.

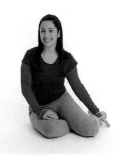

Fern Berenberg has been a Pilates student for five years. Before that, her only exercise routine was "Virtual Aerobics" ... she watched people exercise and imagined herself doing the same. Now she works out regularly and is, in her own words, a "Pilates addict."

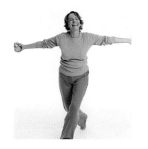

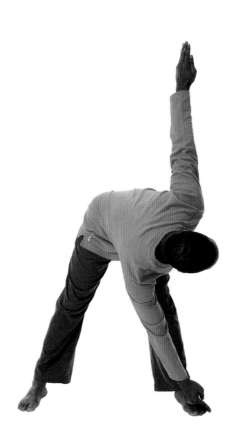